The Extraction of Teeth

The Extraction of Teeth

Second edition
Third Revised Reprint

Geoffrey L Howe
TD, MDS (Dunelm), MRCS (Eng),
LRCP (Lond), FDS RCS (Eng),
FFD RCS (Ire)

Professor of Oral Surgery and Oral Medicine,
Dean, Faculty of Dentistry,
Jordan University of Science and Technology, Irbid, Jordan
formerly Professor of Oral Surgery,
Royal Dental Hospital of London, School of Dental Surgery
(University of London)

wright

Wright
An imprint of Butterworth-Heinemann
Linacre House, Jordan Hill, Oxford OX2 8DP
A division of Reed Educational and Professional Publishing Ltd

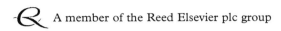 A member of the Reed Elsevier plc group

OXFORD   BOSTON   JOHANNESBURG
MELBOURNE   NEW DELHI   SINGAPORE

First published 1961
Second edition 1970
Revised reprint 1974
Reprinted 1977
Revised reprint 1980
Reprinted 1983, 1987
Revised reprint 1990
Reprinted 1994, 1996

British Library Cataloguing in Publication Data
Howe, Geoffrey Leslie
    The extraction of teeth 2nd ed
    1. Teeth extraction
    I. Title
    617.6′6   RK531

ISBN 0 7236 2231 0

Printed and bound in Great Britain at the University Press, Cambridge

PREFACE TO THE SECOND EDITION

THE reception accorded to the Second Edition of this little book since its appearance a relatively short time ago has led me to make only minor alterations in this revised reprint. The work remains an introductory text and as such is intended to be complementary to *Minor Oral Surgery* and *Local Anaesthesia in Dentistry*. The decision to adhere to this policy was only reached after a considerable amount of thought and discussion with a number of colleagues to whom I am indebted. I am particularly grateful to Professor David Poswillo (Royal College of Surgeons of England) for his thoughtful and constructive criticisms. Fig. 31 was kindly provided by Surgical Equipment Supplies Ltd. whilst Fig. 60 is used by the courtesy of Mr. M. A. Young.

G. L. H.

London
April, 1974

PREFACE TO THE FIRST EDITION

THE student can become a proficient extractor of teeth only with practice. However, before he extracts his first tooth it is essential that he should understand the basic principles underlying the techniques which he must employ. The sole aim of this book is to help him to acquire this fundamental knowledge and the omission of chapters dealing with such topics as the removal of impacted mandibular third molars and oral surgery under endotracheal anaesthesia is deliberate. He must also possess the requisite knowledge of anatomy and local and general anaesthesia, subjects outside the scope of this small volume. Clarity and brevity are essential in any book designed to aid beginners, and so I have attempted to emphasize basic principles and to avoid extolling the virtues of particular instruments and making comparisons between different techniques. The student should remember that there are usually several ways of doing anything well, and that until he has mastered one technique he lacks a yardstick against which to measure the merits or demerits of others.

Throughout this work I have assumed that the operator is right-handed. Left-handed operators must reverse sides in the relevant portions of the text.

This book would not have been written without the encouragement, advice, and assistance of many colleagues at the Eastman and Newcastle upon Tyne Dental Hospitals. I am indebted to each and every one of them. Mr. D. P. Hammersley has been responsible for all the line drawings and the entire text has been read, criticized, and improved by Sir William Kelsey Fry, Mr. P. Bradnum, and Mr. L. W. Kay.

Finally, I would like to dedicate this book to two of my friends and teachers, Mr. T. Stretton and Mr. H. W. Breese, who had so much patience with me when I was a struggling beginner in the art of tooth extraction.

G. L. H.

Newcastle upon Tyne
April, 1961

CONTENTS

FOREWORD TO THE FIRST EDITION

By the late Sir William Kelsey Fry, C.B.E., M.C.

ALTHOUGH the extraction of teeth is one of the oldest and most frequently performed of surgical operations, little has been written concerning simple extractions compared with the mass of literature on the removal of difficult teeth, such as impactions. The author has done a valuable service to both undergraduates and postgraduates in pointing out the need to understand the basic principles underlying the techniques for the removal of individual teeth. For every tooth there is an easy 'back-door' method of extraction and these methods are clearly outlined in this book. I am particularly pleased to see the insistence on the necessity of using sharp forceps, which are so essential for efficient extractions.

The need for preoperative assessment and postoperative care is another aspect of extraction which is often neglected. The author's insistence on its importance is another feature of a book which, in my opinion, will prove of considerable value to all those who are not too proud to learn something new of the art of simple extraction.

THE EXTRACTION OF TEETH

CHAPTER I

INTRODUCTION

Tooth Extraction.—The *ideal* tooth extraction is the painless removal of the whole tooth, or tooth-root, with minimal trauma to the investing tissues, so that the wound heals uneventfully and no postoperative prosthetic problem is created.

The dental surgeon should endeavour to make every tooth extraction he performs an ideal one, and in order to attain this objective he must adapt his technique to deal with the difficulties and possible complications presented by the extraction of each individual tooth.

Indications for tooth extraction may be many and varied. If conservative treatment has either failed or is not indicated, a tooth may have to be extracted because of either periodontal disease, caries, periapical infection, erosion, abrasion, attrition, hypoplasia, or pulpal lesions (e.g., pulpitis, 'pink spot' or pulpal hyperplasia).

Trauma to the teeth or jaws may cause dislocation of a tooth from its socket. More commonly, either the root or crown of the tooth is fractured or the tooth is partially dislocated from its socket. Any of these accidents may necessitate extraction of the damaged tooth. More severe trauma may cause a fractured jaw, and in these circumstances it is often necessary to remove a tooth lying in the fracture line. Sometimes a healthy, sound tooth must be extracted as part of an overall orthodontic or prosthetic treatment plan, or before starting a course of therapeutic irradiation.

Basically only two *methods* of extraction are available. The first method, which suffices in most cases, is usually called 'forceps extraction', and consists of removing the tooth or root by the use of forceps or elevators or both. The blades of these instruments are forced down the periodontal membrane between the tooth-root and the bony socket wall, none of which is removed electively. This method is better described as *intra-alveolar* extraction, and is described in Chapter II.

The other method of extraction is to dissect the tooth or root from its bony attachments. This separation is achieved by removal of some of the bone investing the roots, which are then delivered by the use of elevators and/or forceps. This technique is commonly called the 'surgical method', but as all extractions, however performed, are surgical procedures, a better and more accurate name would be *trans-alveolar* extraction (*see* Chapter III).

The Mechanical Principles of Extraction.—The three mechanical principles of extraction are:—

1. *Expansion of the bony socket* to permit the removal of its contained tooth. This is achieved by using the tooth as the dilating instrument, and is the most important factor in 'forceps extraction'.

To be successful it requires that sufficient tooth be present to be firmly grasped by the forceps blades. The root pattern of the tooth must be such that it is possible to dilate the socket sufficiently to permit the complete dislocation of the tooth from its socket (*Fig.* 1). The socket can be dilated only if the bone of which it is composed is sufficiently elastic to permit such

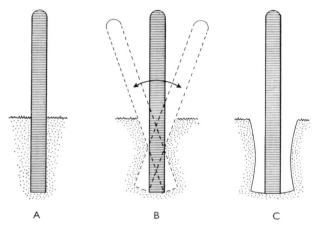

A   B   C

Fig. 1.—The removal of a post embedded in the ground (A) is performed by moving the post laterally (B) until the earth surrounding it has been displaced sufficiently (C) to permit the post to be lifted out. A tooth is removed in a similar fashion when forceps are used although the conical shape of the tooth-root and the consistency of the bone enclosing it combine to limit or even prevent lateral movement of the apex.

expansion. This property is maximal in young bone and decreases with age. In most cases dilatation of the socket is accompanied by multiple small fractures of the buccal plate and the inter-radicular septa. These bony fragments usually retain their periosteal attachment and should be replaced by digital compression at the completion of the extraction. All loose bony fragments which have lost more than half of their periosteal attachment should be removed from the wound because their blood-supply will be so impaired that they will die. The presence of a devitalized bony fragment is a pre-disposing cause of post-extraction haemorrhage, delayed healing, and wound infection until exfoliation occurs. The value and importance of débridement following tooth extraction cannot be overemphasized.

If the root pattern or consistency of the investing bone is such that the dilatation of the socket is impracticable, then the *trans-alveolar* method of extraction, with or without the division of the roots of multi-rooted teeth, must be employed.

2. *The use of a lever and fulcrum* to force a tooth or root out of the socket along the path of least resistance. This is the basic factor governing the use of elevators to extract teeth and roots, and the use of these instruments is described on pages 34 to 36.

3. *The insertion of a wedge or wedges* between the tooth-root and the bony socket wall, thus causing the tooth to rise in its socket (*Fig.* 2). In most cases this factor can be disregarded owing to the elasticity of the investing alveolar bone. It does, however, explain why some conically rooted mandibular premolars and molars sometimes 'shoot' out of their sockets when forceps blades are applied to them.

Preoperative Assessment.—Good preoperative assessment of difficulties which may be encountered or complications which may occur is the basis of successful extraction technique. Time spent in making a careful preoperative assessment is never wasted!

A *history* of general disease, nervousness, resistance to inhalation anaesthesia, or previous difficulty with extractions, will govern both the choice of anaesthesia (*see* p. 10) and the method used to deliver the tooth. While the history is being taken, a general impression of the patient is formed and the size of his mouth and jaws noted. The general cleanliness of the patient's mouth and the efficiency of his oral hygiene are then observed. Wherever necessary and whenever possible, a careful *pre-extraction scaling* should be performed, especially in neglected mouths, at least one week prior to surgery being undertaken.

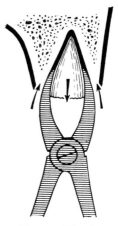

Fig. 2.—The insertion of the wedge-shaped forceps blades may cause the tooth to rise in its socket.

Calculus, stagnation, and chronic inflammation usually occur together, and local healing processes may be delayed unless the mouth is thoroughly cleaned prior to the removal of teeth. It is also possible for the patient to inhale fragments of tartar or other infected material during the extraction, especially when the surgery is performed under general anaesthesia in the dental chair. Such a mishap may cause a pulmonary infection.

Painstaking *clinical examination* of the tooth to be extracted and its supporting structures always yields valuable information. The tooth may be heavily restored or grossly carious, inclined or rotated, firm or mobile, while supporting structures may be either diseased or hypertrophied. The accessibility of the tooth and the amount and site of sound tooth-substance remaining should be carefully noted. Teeth with shallow, broad crowns often have long roots, whilst those which exhibit marked attrition usually have calcified pulp chambers and are brittle. Such teeth are often set in dense unyielding bone,

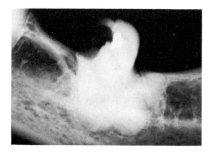

Fig. 3.—The extraction of this hyper-cementosed lower molar had been un-successfully attempted with forceps. The retained root is evidence of previous difficulty with extractions.

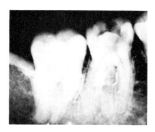

Fig. 4.—This mandibular first molar proved resistant to forceps extraction. A radiograph revealed the presence of three roots.

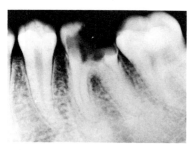

Fig. 5.—It was decided to remove this broken-down pulpless mandibular first molar by dissection. A pre-extraction radiograph revealed its unfavourable root pattern and the presence of sclerosis of the alveolar bone enclosing the roots.

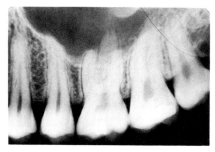

Fig. 6.—A maxillary first permanent molar with widely splayed roots in intimate relationship with the maxillary antrum.

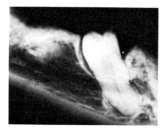

Fig. 7.—The root of this unerupted distally inclined mandibular second pre-molar is grooved by the inferior dental nerve and close to the mental foramen.

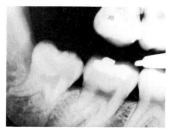

Fig. 8.—A four-rooted mandibular third molar which resisted forceps extraction.

the outer plate of which has a convex surface. Pulpless teeth may have resorbed roots and are often rather fragile.

In many instances a complete *preoperative* assessment can only be made if the clinical examination is supplemented by a *pre-extraction radiograph*. It is not usually practicable to take a preoperative radiograph before every extraction, but one should always be taken if any of the following positive indications exist.

Indications for a Preoperative Radiograph.—

1. A history of difficult or attempted extractions (*Fig.* 3).

2. A tooth which is abnormally resistant to forceps extraction (*Figs.* 4, 8, 16).

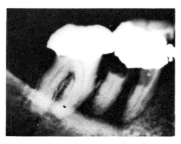

Fig. 9.—A heavily restored and carious mandibular molar.

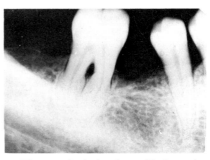

Fig. 10.—An isolated mandibular molar affected by periodontal disease involving the bifurcation showing sclerosis of bone and hypercementosis of roots.

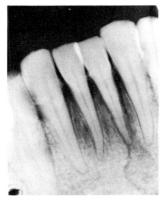

Fig. 11.—A mandibular incisor in the line of an undisplaced fracture of the mandible.

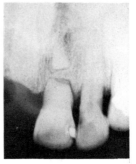

Fig. 12.—An incisor, the root of which had been fractured many years before this radiograph was taken. The pulp chamber and canal are obliterated and the apical portion is separated from the remainder of the root by a bony barrier.

3. If, after clinical examination, it has been decided to remove the tooth by dissection (*Fig.* 5).

4. Any teeth or roots in close relationship to either the maxillary antrum or the inferior dental and mental nerves (*Figs.* 6, 7).

5. All mandibular third molars, instanding premolars, or misplaced canines (*Fig.* 8). The root pattern of such teeth is often abnormal.

6. Heavily restored or pulpless teeth. These teeth are normally very brittle (*Figs.* 9, 14).

7. Any tooth affected by periodontal disease accompanied by some sclerosis of the supporting bone. Such teeth are often hypercementosed and brittle (*Fig.* 10).

8. Any tooth which has been subjected to trauma. Fractures of the roots and/or alveolar bone may be present (*Figs.* 11, 12).

9. An isolated maxillary molar, especially if it is unopposed and over-erupted (*Figs.* 13, 16). The bony support of such a tooth is often weakened

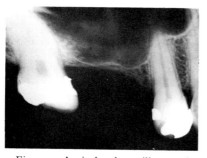

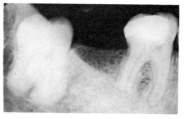

Fig. 13.—An isolated maxillary molar, the bony support of which is weakened by the presence of a large maxillary antrum.

Fig. 14.—A partially erupted mandibular third molar with hypercementosed roots. The first molar is heavily restored, pulpless, and its distal root is resorbed.

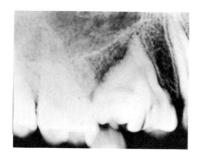

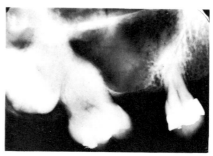

Fig. 15.—A gemination in the maxillary premolar region.

Fig. 16.—A pathological gemination between an unerupted maxillary third molar and an isolated maxillary second molar. Note the large antrum.

by the presence of a large maxillary antrum. This may predispose to either the creation of an oro-antral communication or fracture of the maxillary tuberosity.

10. Any partially erupted or unerupted tooth or retained root (*Fig.* 14).

11. Any tooth whose abnormal crown or delayed eruption might indicate the possibility of dilaceration, gemination, or a dilated odontome (*Figs.* 15, 16).

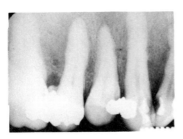 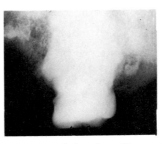

Fig. 17.—Generalized hypercementosis in osteitis deformans (Paget's disease of bone).

Fig. 18.—An ankylosed maxillary molar in a patient with osteitis deformans.

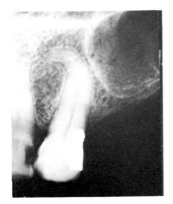 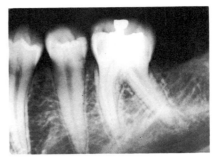

Fig. 19.—A maxillary canine with a hooked root in close relationship to the maxillary antrum.

Fig. 20.—A mandibular molar with widely splayed roots.

12. Any condition which predisposes to dental or alveolar abnormality, e.g.:—

a. Osteitis deformans in which the roots are hypercementosed and there is a predisposition to chronic osteomyelitis (*Figs.* 17, 18).

b. Cleido-cranial dysostosis, for pseudo-anodontia and hooked roots occur in this condition.

c. Patients who have received therapeutic irradiation to the jaws and thus have a predisposition to osteoradionecrosis.

d. Osteopetrosis, which causes extractions to be difficult and predisposes to chronic osteomyelitis.

Requirements of a Pre-extraction Radiograph.—A pre-extraction radiograph must show the whole root structure and the alveolar bone investing the tooth. In most cases an intra-oral periapical view will suffice, but sometimes an extra-oral lateral oblique view of the mandible will be required to demonstrate the entire root, or the state, structure, and amount of supporting bone.

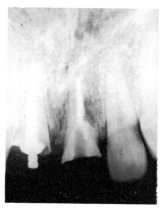 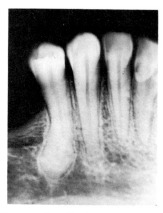

Fig. 21.—A replanted maxillary central incisor showing marked resorption of the root.

Fig. 22.—Localized hypercementosis.

A good radiograph is wasted unless it is carefully interpreted. The use of a hand lens and viewing box greatly aid interpretation and enable the following *factors causing difficulty* to be detected:—

1. Abnormal number of roots (*Figs.* 4, 8).
2. Abnormal shape of roots (*Fig.* 19).
3. An unfavourable root pattern (*Figs.* 3, 5, 20).
4. Caries extending into the root or root-mass (*Fig.* 9).
5. Fracture or resorption of the root (*Figs.* 12, 21).
6. Hypercementosis of roots (*Figs.* 3, 10, 14, 17, 18, 22, 23).
7. Ankylosis (*Figs.* 18, 24).
8. Geminations (*Figs.* 15, 16).
9. Impacted teeth (*Fig.* 25).
10. Bony sclerosis and pathological lesions (*Fig.* 26).

While it is easy to diagnose areas of localized bony sclerosis on a radiograph (*Fig.* 27), an accurate assessment of generalized bony sclerosis is only possible if both exposure and developing technique are carefully standardized. A less accurate, though useful, guide is based upon the size of the cancellous bone-spaces shown in the radiograph. Large spaces are usually found in elastic, yielding bone (*Figs.* 6, 19, 20, 25) while small spaces surrounded by thick, radio-opaque trabeculae characterize sclerotic bone (*Figs.* 5, 21, 24).

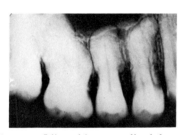

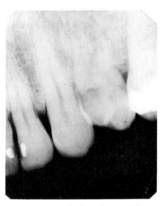

Fig. 23.—Idiopathic generalized hyper-cementosis.

Fig. 24.—An ankylosed maxillary first premolar.

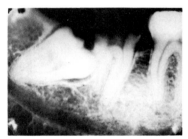

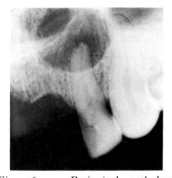

Fig. 25.—The lower right second molar resisted extraction with forceps and its crown was fractured. This radiograph reveals that an unerupted mandibular third molar was impacted into the tooth.

Fig. 26. — Periapical pathological lesions may be retained when the tooth is extracted unless diagnosed preoperatively. This dental cyst was discovered in a patient who had received dental treatment regularly for many years.

Careful interpretation of the radiograph may also reveal the possibility of the following *complications*:—

1. Involvement of, and damage to, the inferior dental and mental nerves (*Fig.* 7).

2. The creation of an oro-antral or oronasal communication (*Figs.* 6, 13).

3. The retention of intra-bony pathological lesions (*Fig.* 26).

4. The displacement of a tooth or root into the maxillary antrum (*Figs.* 6, 13).

5. Fracture of the maxillary tuberosity (*Figs.* 13, 16).

Once the difficulties and possible complications have been diagnosed, the method of extraction to be used for the removal of the tooth under consideration can be decided, and the type of anaesthesia to be employed must then be considered.

The terms 'analgesia' and 'anaesthesia' are often used quite incorrectly as if they were synonymous. *Analgesia* is loss of pain sensation without loss of other forms of sensation (e.g., temperature and pressure). *Anaesthesia* is loss of all forms of consciousness, and is often accompanied by loss of motor function.

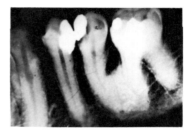

Fig. 27.—Localized bony sclerosis of unknown aetiology.

Anaesthesia or analgesia may affect a part of the body only and is then described as *local* anaesthesia or analgesia. If the whole body is affected the term *general* anaesthesia or analgesia is applied. Anaesthesia is preferable to analgesia when teeth are being extracted.

Choice of Anaesthesia.—Teeth may be extracted under either local or general anaesthesia and the dental surgeon must assess the indications and contra-indications of both before deciding which to use in a particular case. On many occasions either method will suffice, and in these circumstances the patient may be allowed to choose between them. However, if there is a positive contra-indication to the method of anaesthesia for which the patient has a preference, the dental surgeon should not be persuaded to use a technique which is not in the best interests of his patient, but should follow the dictates of his trained opinion. Modern anaesthesia is such that specialist anaesthetists with full hospital facilities seldom, if ever, refuse to give a general anaesthetic to an in-patient, however unfit he may be, provided that such an anaesthetic is administered for an absolutely essential procedure. These facilities are neither available nor necessary for routine dental extractions, and the type of general anaesthesia discussed here is that induced in an out-patient in the dental chair.

Hurry is the enemy of good oral surgery and an ill-chosen form of anaesthesia is a common cause of hurry. The dental surgeon should learn to estimate with accuracy the time required to complete each extraction. This enables him to choose a form of anaesthesia which will provide adequate operating time for the completion of his task. A good dental anaesthetist can usually provide 5 to 10 minutes' operating time under a general anaesthetic of inhalational type in the dental chair without the risk of anoxia or other complications. Although some exceptionally experienced and skilled anaesthetists are able to double this operating time, as a general rule the dental surgeon should not choose this form of anaesthesia for any operation which is likely to last for more than 5 minutes. Local anaesthesia may be used for any dental operation of 30 to 45 minutes' duration, but any extraction needing longer than this is an indication for admission to hospital and the administration of an endotracheal general anaesthetic.

Both general and local factors govern the choice of anaesthesia for the extraction of a particular tooth, and the operator must be fully conversant with them if he is to make a correct choice.

General Factors governing the Choice of Anaesthesia.—Very large or very obese patients are often unsuitable subjects for a general anaesthetic in the dental chair, especially if they have any tendency towards alcoholism. The co-operation of the patient is not only essential when local anaesthesia is being employed, but it can be used to great advantage to facilitate the extraction. Some patients are incapable of this co-operation for such reasons as fear, apprehension, extreme nervousness, hysteria, mental deficiency, or insanity. Young children below the age of reason find it impossible to distinguish between pressure and pain and so are liable to prove unco-operative if local anaesthesia is used. In some instances the judicious use of premedication may make the employment of local anaesthesia possible, but in most cases extraction of teeth for these patients is easier if general anaesthesia is used. The induction of general anaesthesia in these cases may be difficult, and may tax to the full both the skill and patience of the most experienced dental anaesthetist. Epileptics are usually good subjects for either local or general anaesthesia provided that they have not omitted to take the anticonvulsive drugs to which they are accustomed and anoxia is avoided.

Systemic disease may be the deciding factor which influences the choice of anaesthesia. Any disease which impairs either respiratory efficiency or the patency of the airway is a contra-indication to general anaesthesia in the dental chair. Chronic bronchitis, emphysema, bronchiectasis, asthma, tuberculosis, and excessive smoking interfere with respiratory exchanges, while nasal obstruction, paralysis of the vocal cords, and space-occupying lesions of the neck may interfere with the patency of the airway. Any acute infection of the respiratory tract is an absolute contra-indication to general anaesthesia in the dental chair, and in these cases local anaesthesia should be employed if the extraction cannot be postponed. Acute infection in the floor of the mouth is a contra-indication to any form of anaesthesia in an out-patient. Oedema of the glottis and laryngeal obstruction may complicate general anaesthesia in such circumstances, while local anaesthesia is impracticable. These patients should be admitted to hospital and any necessary surgery performed under endotracheal anaesthesia. Patients afflicted with either anaemia, especially sickle-cell disease and trait, or cardiovascular disease do not withstand anoxia or hypotension well, however temporary it may be. For this reason it is better to employ local anaesthesia in these cases whenever it is practicable to do so. While some authorities advise the omission of adrenaline from the local anaesthetic solutions administered to patients suffering from cardiovascular disease, opinion is prevalent that the small amounts of adrenaline administered for dental purposes are, in fact, beneficial, because they ensure a more certain, prolonged, and profound anaesthesia and thus decrease the amount of adrenaline secreted by the patient himself in response to pain or fear. *It is important that any extraction or scaling performed on a patient suffering from either congenital or rheumatic valvular heart disease should be undertaken only with adequate antibiotic cover.* In some centres, patients with ischaemic heart disease who have had a cardiac infarct are treated in the same way. Patients afflicted with severe heart disease should be admitted to hospital for dental extractions whatever form of anaesthesia is to be used.

Many anaesthetists prefer not to administer a general anaesthetic in the dental chair to a woman in the first or last three months of pregnancy, as they fear that any anoxic episode during the anaesthetic may damage the foetus. Pregnancy is not a contra-indication to the use of local anaesthesia, which, however, should not be used in certain rare haemorrhagic diseases such as haemophilia, Christmas disease, or von Willebrand's disease, owing to the risk of bleeding at the injection site and the needle track. The dangers associated with dental extractions in these patients are such as to make admission to hospital and full haematological cover imperative. In general, the patient classified as a poor anaesthetic risk should be treated as an in-patient under either local anaesthesia or endotracheal anaesthesia. However, patients afflicted with thyrotoxicosis are especially susceptible to adverse reactions to adrenaline.

Until comparatively recent times most local anaesthetic agents available for use in dental surgery contained the *p*-aminobenzoic acid ring. This molecular structure is also found in certain other drugs (e.g., sulphonamides) and some patients acquire a sensitivity to it. The administration of any substance which contains this ring in its molecule (e.g., procaine or benzocaine) is contra-indicated in sensitized subjects (*Fig.* 28). Fortunately, the introduction of lignocaine (lidocaine, Xylocaine), and prilocaine (Citanest), local anaesthetic agents with a completely different chemical structure, has made it possible to utilize an alternative agent when the patient either gives a history of or exhibits sensitivity to a particular drug.

Certain practical considerations may govern our choice of anaesthesia. *A dental surgeon should never attempt to administer a general anaesthetic and extract teeth at the same time.* If a dental anaesthetist is not available he should use local anaesthesia if this is possible. The techniques of local anaesthesia are easily mastered, the equipment required is limited in amount, economical, and easily transportable. No preoperative preparation of the patient is required for local anaesthesia, and the patient can leave the surgery unescorted and often return to work after local anaesthesia has been used.

Local Factors governing the Choice of Anaesthesia.—The most important contra-indication to local anaesthesia is the presence of acute infection at the site of operation. Injections of local anaesthetic solution into acutely inflamed areas spread the infection and seldom produce anaesthesia. It is sometimes possible to use regional anaesthesia to obtain the desired effect, but no attempt should be made to use a mandibular block in patients with infections in the floor of the mouth or retromolar area (*see* p. 11). If it is desirable

PROCAINE

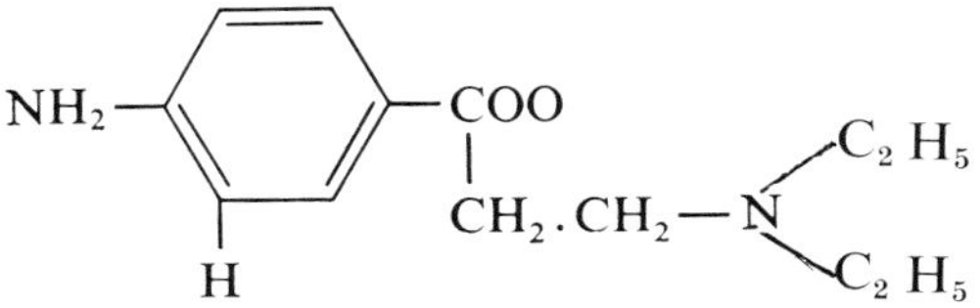

NH_2—⟨ring⟩—COO
        |
        $CH_2.CH_2$—N⟨$C_2 H_5$ / $C_2 H_5$⟩
H

SULPHONAMIDE

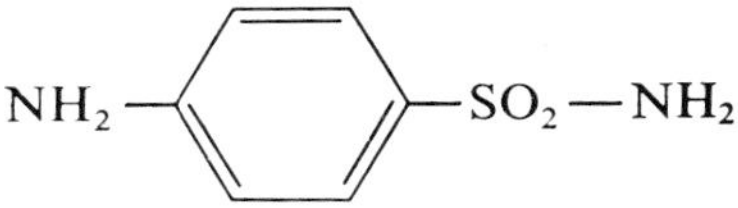

NH_2—⟨ring⟩—SO_2—NH_2

LIGNOCAINE

CH_3
⟨ring⟩—NH—CO—CH_2—N⟨$C_2 H_5$ / $C_2 H_5$⟩
CH_3

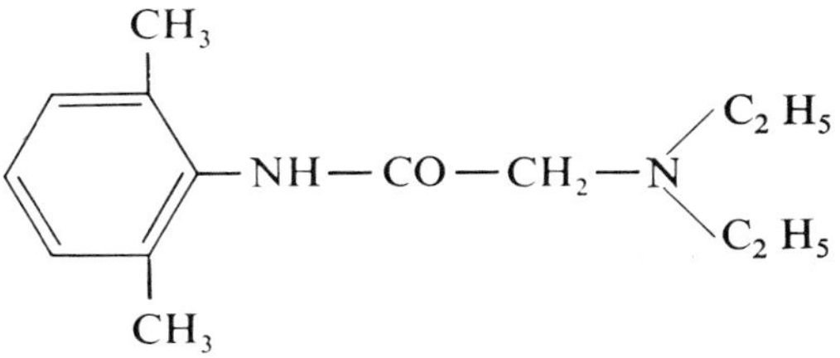

Fig. 28.—Although chemically related to procaine and sulphonamide, lignocaine does not contain the *p*-amino group which seems to be responsible for inducing allergic sensitivity.

to extract several teeth in varying quadrants of the mouth in one sitting, the necessity for multiple injections may make the use of local anaesthesia undesirable and general anaesthesia preferable. The vasoconstrictor contained in most local anaesthetic solutions assists haemostasis thus providing a drier field of operation for the surgeon. The operating time available for haemostasis under local anaesthesia may indicate its use in patients with a history of post-extraction haemorrhage, in whom the presence of an underlying haemorrhagic disease has been excluded. If the tendency to bleed is due to the presence of a local abnormality, such as a haemangioma, local anaesthesia should be avoided and the extraction undertaken only in hospital with full haematological facilities. The blood-supply of any bone which has received therapeutic irradiation is impaired, and the use of local anaesthesia with its contained vasoconstrictor is contra-indicated for the extraction of teeth in these cases owing to the risk of osteoradionecrosis supervening.

Of necessity, the many contra-indications, advantages, and disadvantages of local and general anaesthesia in the dental chair have been emphasized. It is of great importance to remember that both methods have been in widespread use for a long time, and that the morbidity is infinitesimal if care is taken in the selection of the appropriate method. The dental surgeon should make careful inquiries about the general medical history of any patient consulting him, and in cases of difficulty he should enlist the aid of the patient's physician before selecting the form of anaesthesia to be employed.

It is also important to make inquiries about current drug therapy because some drugs prescribed for the treatment of systemic disease may interact with those used for anaesthetic purposes. Many patients are unaware of the name or nature of medicines they are taking. For this reason if doubt exists the dentist should contact the doctor concerned to ascertain details of the medication before proceeding with dental treatment. At the same time he should also receive guidance concerning the severity of the systemic condition and its relationship to dental treatment.

Table 1.—Some Tricyclic Anti-depressive Drugs

Official Name	*Proprietary Names*
Amitriptyline	Amizol, Domical, Larozyl (Sweden), Limbitrol (also contains chlordiazepoxide), Saroten, Triptafen, and Tryptizol
Clomipramine	Anafranil
Desipramine	Pertofran
Imipramine	Berkomine, Tofranil, Praminil, Norpramine, Impril (Canada), Imiprin (Australia), Iramil
Nortriptyline	Allegron, Aventyl; Motipress and Motival are compound preparations of nortriptyline and fluphenazine
Opipramol	Insidon
Protriptyline	Concordin
Trimipramine	Surmontil

In recent years the treatment of depressive illness has been revolutionized by the introduction of the monoamine oxidase inhibitor and tricyclic drugs. When the former were first introduced it was thought that they would potentiate the action of adrenaline or noradrenaline to provoke a dangerous rise in blood-pressure. In the light of experience it is now accepted that the small amounts of amine vasoconstrictors contained in local anaesthetic solutions do not constitute any danger to dental patients taking this type of drug.

Greater caution must be exercised if local anaesthesia is required for patients taking any of the tricyclic group of anti-depressive drugs (*Table 1*), which are also used to treat nocturnal enuresis in children. It has been demonstrated that the effects of noradrenaline are potentiated significantly by drugs of the tricyclic group and the effects of adrenaline to a lesser extent. These vasoconstrictors should not be injected in patients taking tricyclic anti-depressive drugs because of the risk of producing hypertension or cardiac arrhythmia. Either local anaesthetic solutions that do not contain adrenaline or noradrenaline, or a prilocaine preparation containing felypressin, a non-amine vasoconstrictor (Citanest with Octapressin), should be used under these circumstances.

A profound hypertensive reaction is characterized by the sudden onset of a severe headache. Whilst this phenomenon is usually transient, it may be complicated by either intracranial haemorrhage or acute heart failure. These complications may be avoided by the intramuscular or intravenous injection of 5 mg. phentolamine (Rogitine), but as such treatment may produce a labile blood-pressure it is best carried out by experts with the aid of electronic monitoring equipment. For this reason any patient exhibiting such a reaction should be transferred to hospital without delay.

Occasionally a dentist performing surgery under general anaesthesia may wish to use a solution containing a vasoconstrictor in order to reduce the vascularity of the operative site. If so, he should always consult the anaesthetist prior to the induction of anaesthesia, for adrenaline or noradrenaline may provoke cardiac arrhythmia when used in conjunction with such agents as halothane, ethyl chloride, trichlorethylene, and cyclopropane. There is no evidence that felypressin produces a similar complication, so that prilocaine with felypressin may be used safely under these circumstances. However it is a less effective vasoconstrictor.

Although procaine is now seldom employed in dentistry it should be noted that this local anaesthetic agent should not be used in patients receiving sulphonamides for the treatment of systemic disease. As this group of antibacterial drugs contains the same para-amino benzoic acid ring as procaine, it is theoretically possible that they could partially neutralize the effects of each other if administered concurrently. Although this phenomenon has never been proved clinically, the combination is better avoided. Patients who give a history of hypersensitivity to sulphonamides should not receive a local anaesthetic agent containing the para-amino benzoic acid ring. (*Fig* 28, p. 13.)

Sterilization.—Many diseases are caused by infection with microorganisms, and those micro-organisms which cause disease are described as being *pathogenic*. If pathogenic micro-organisms are introduced into an operation wound there is a serious risk that the wound will break down and healing will be delayed. The surgeon attempts to prevent the occurrence of this undesirable postoperative complication by using aseptic techniques and by sterilizing the instruments and materials used during the operation. *Sterilization* may be defined as the removal of all micro-organisms from a given object, or their effective destruction, whilst *asepsis* is a method of surgery which is designed to prevent the introduction of infection into a wound at the time of operation or when wounds are dressed.

The healthy mouth is heavily contaminated with micro-organisms of many types, some of which are potentially pathogenic. It is quite impossible to render the mouth sterile, although the number of micro-organisms present can be reduced considerably by attention to oral hygiene and pre-extraction scaling of the teeth. Despite every care being taken it is still necessary to operate in a non-sterile field, and it is fortunate that the oral tissues appear to have especially efficient defensive mechanisms which usually deal with the contamination of the wound which inevitably occurs. Although coping successfully with autogenous infection, these defences are more vulnerable to micro-organisms introduced into the mouth from other sources at the time of operation, so that the hands of the operator should be thoroughly cleansed and instruments sterilized before use. The operator should keep his finger-nails short and clean, and the hands should be scrubbed with soap and water and dried upon a clean towel immediately before performing a dental extraction or any other intra-oral surgery.

In order to kill the most resistant micro-organisms, namely, bacterial spores, it is necessary either to subject them to moist heat at 120° C. for 10 to 12 minutes in an *autoclave* or steam pressure sterilizer, or to dry heat at 160° C. for 60 minutes in a *hot-air oven*. Water boils at 100° C. at normal temperature and pressure, and bacterial spores may resist these conditions for 60 minutes and fungi and thread organisms for 20 minutes. Therefore hot water 'sterilization' cannot produce complete sterility and as this form of disinfection is still widely employed in general dental practice it is fortunate that the majority of pathogenic bacteria which may be present are in the vegetative phase and are destroyed by immersion in *boiling* water for 5 to 10 minutes. The limitations of the method make careful technique essential if a breakdown of sterility is not to occur. The instruments must be thoroughly washed and all blood, pus, and other debris removed from them. All the instruments should be completely submerged so that their entire surface area is in contact with boiling water. *After boiling point has been regained* the instruments should be boiled for a minimum of 5 minutes, and during this time no other instruments must be added to the load in the hot water bath. When the period of boiling is complete the instruments are transferred with sterile Cheatle forceps to trays containing a chemical sterilizing agent until required for use. Most chemical sterilizing agents do not make an instrument completely sterile, but immersion in 70 per cent ethyl alcohol with 0·075 per cent chlorhexidine digluconate and 0·75 per cent Cetrimide B.P. for 30 minutes will kill vegetative micro-organisms, and these agents are useful for maintaining the 'sterility' of instruments previously disinfected by boiling.

Homologous serum jaundice is a disease caused by the virus of serum hepatitis known as 'Virus B' which some healthy people harbour in their blood for prolonged periods, even perhaps indefinitely, without exhibiting any clinical symptoms or signs of viral hepatitis. However, if this virus is transmitted from such an individual to one who is susceptible to it the full manifestations of viral hepatitis may be produced. Patients contracting infective hepatitis as a result of treatment by their dentists are rarely seen by them because the incubation period may be as long as 160 days. By this time the patient does not associate his condition with dental treatment and consults his doctor. In dental practice the risk of cross-infection is greatest if inadequately sterilized syringes and needles are used. A Medical Research Council report published in 1962 contained a reference to the admission to one hospital during a two-year period of 15 cases, 3 of which were fatal, following dental procedures. The high risk of transmission of this dangerous disease during dental procedures is the reason why a hypodermic needle should never be used on more than one patient. The Report of the Expert Group on Hepatitis in Dentistry—published in January, 1979 by Her Majesty's Stationery Office—gives guidance on the dental management of such patients.

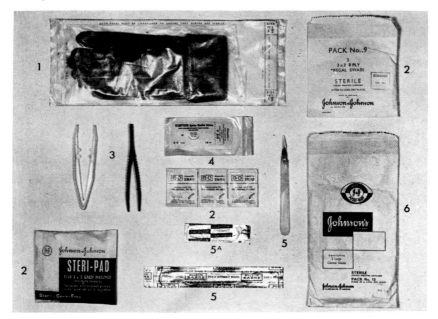

Fig. 29.—Sterile disposable surgical equipment. 1, Gloves; 2, Swabs; 3, Dressing tweezers; 4, Sutures; 5, Scalpel handle; 5A, Scalpel blades; 6, Towels.

The general dental practitioner who intends to undertake any appreciable amount of oral surgery has a duty to maintain a standard of both sterilization and asepsis which is above the average level. This can often be achieved by the use of sterilized disposable equipment and dressings (*Fig.* 29), a reasonably priced hot-air oven (*Fig.* 30), and a completely automatic high-speed instrument autoclave such as the type illustrated in *Fig.* 31. No endeavour should be spared to exclude extraneous bacteria from the operative site, even though it is not possible to achieve a standard of asepsis comparable with that maintained in the operating theatre of a modern hospital.

Major items of dental equipment such as engines, lights, and chairs are inevitably a source of cross-infection and for this reason any necessary adjustments to them should be made, whenever possible, by an assistant who is not participating in the operation. Should circumstances preclude this, a sterile clothes peg or a piece of sterile gauze should be used to prevent contamination when any alteration in the position of the operating light is required. Cable engine arms should be enclosed within a sterile tube of gauze throughout the operation.

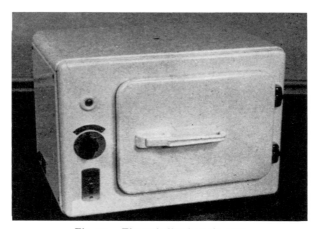

Fig. 30.—Electrohelios hot-air oven.

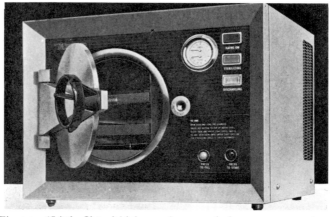

Fig. 31.—'Little Sister' high-speed automatic instrument autoclave.

General Arrangements.—

Position of the Operator.—When extracting any tooth except the right mandibular molars, premolars, and canines, the operator stands on the right-hand side of the patient as shown in *Fig.* 32 A. For the removal of right mandibular cheek teeth by the intra-alveolar method, the operator stands behind the patient as shown in *Fig.* 32 C. Sometimes the operator must stand upon a raised platform or 'operating box' in order to achieve the optimal working position.

Height of the Dental Chair.—This is an important consideration which is often ignored. If the site of the operation is either too high or too low in

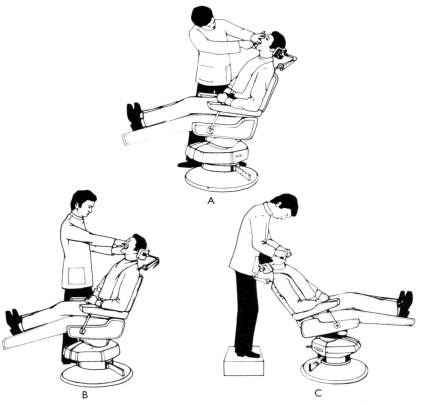

Fig. 32.—Position of the operator during the extraction of: A, All teeth except the right mandibular cheek teeth. B, The left mandibular cheek teeth. C, The right mandibular cheek teeth.

relation to the operator, he works at a mechanical disadvantage and in a tiring and uncomfortable position.

When a maxillary tooth is being extracted, the chair should be adjusted so that the site of operation is about 8 cm. (3 in.) below the shoulder level of the operator (*Fig.* 32 A). During the extraction of a mandibular tooth the chair height should be adjusted so that the tooth to be extracted is about

16 cm. (6 in.) below the level of the operator's elbow (*Fig.* 32 B). When the operator is standing behind the patient (*Fig.* 32 C) the chair should be lowered sufficiently to enable him to have a clear view of the field of operation and to be in a comfortable position while operating. These objectives may be achieved if the dental surgeon uses the 'operating box', especially when dealing with tall patients.

Light.—While it would seem superfluous to state that good illumination of the operative field is an absolute essential for the successful extraction of teeth, failure to ensure adequate lighting of the site of operation is a very common fault, and is the main reason for the failure of a number of attempts at extraction.

The dental surgeon should attempt to acquire a quiet, efficient, unhurried, and methodical approach to his work. This, together with sympathetic encouragement, will do much to gain both the confidence and co-operation of the patient. The operator should avoid increasing the natural misgivings of the patient by displaying instruments only when it is impossible to do otherwise. He should stand with his feet apart during the procedure and must ensure that neither his footwear nor the flooring are such as to impair his balance (*Fig.* 32).

CHAPTER II

INTRA-ALVEOLAR EXTRACTION

The Dental Forceps.—The most widely used instruments employed in the extraction of teeth are the dental forceps. The use of this instrument makes it possible for the operator to grasp the root portion of a tooth and dislocate the latter from its socket by exerting pressure upon it. The simplest and most efficient pattern of dental forceps is the upper straight forceps (*Fig.* 33) and they, like all forceps, have blades and handles united by a hinge joint. The larger the ratio between the length of the handles and the length of the blades the greater the leverage which can be exerted upon the root. The length of the handles must be such that the forceps fit the operator's hand, for the greater the distance between the hinge joint and the operator's hand, the greater is the movement of the forceps within the hand. In this way a great deal of energy may be dissipated.

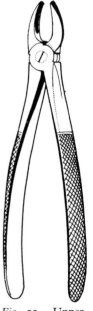

Fig. 33.—Upper straight forceps.

When the forceps are applied to a tooth-root the blades are forced along the periodontal membrane. This is made easier if the forceps blades are really *sharp*, for the sharp blade not only cuts the periodontal fibres cleanly, but also enables the dental surgeon to feel his way along the root surface. Stainless-steel forceps blades can be sharpened with a sandpaper disk applied to the outside of the tips (*Fig.* 34). Ideally, the whole of the inner surface of the forceps blades should fit the root surface (*Fig.* 35 A). In practice the size and shape of roots vary so greatly that it is not possible to achieve this aim, and the root is gripped by the edges of the blades, 'two-point contact' (*Fig.* 35 B). If there is only a single linear contact, 'one-point contact', between root and forceps blade, the tooth will probably be crushed when it is gripped (*Fig.* 35 C). The desirability of achieving 'two-point contact' is an important factor to be considered when selecting the forceps to be used for a particular extraction. It is better to use forceps with blades which are slightly narrow rather than a pair with blades which are too broad. Narrow blades are described as being 'fine' and wide blades are called 'heavy'. Another important principle governing the application of forceps to a tooth is that the long axis of the blades should be either on or parallel to the long axis of the tooth-root. It is easy to apply upper straight forceps in this manner to maxillary incisors and canines, but when an attempt is made to apply them to upper cheek teeth, the lower lip and mandibular incisors

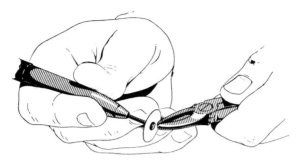

Fig. 34.—Sharpening forceps blades.

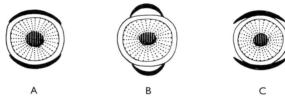

A   B   C

Fig. 35.—Cross-sections of root with forceps blades applied to it. A, Ideal fit. B, 'Two-point contact'. C, 'One-point contact'.

prevent the blades being positioned correctly (Fig. 36 A). In order to overcome this difficulty two bends are introduced into forceps designed for the extraction of maxillary cheek teeth (Fig. 36 B).

Upper premolars have either one root or two roots set side by side (buccal and palatal roots). Thus the blades of upper premolar forceps are 'mirror-images' of each other and the same instrument can be used to extract both right and left maxillary premolars. As the maxillary molars have a single palatal root and two buccal roots, the two blades of the full molar forceps used for the extraction of these teeth are different, the palatal blade being designed to grip one root and the buccal blade designed to grip the mesiobuccal and distobuccal roots above the bifurcation. This difference between the blades, together with the curve of the forceps introduced to avoid the lower lip and ensure their correct application, makes it necessary to have one pair of upper full molar forceps to extract the right maxillary molars and another pair to extract the left.

Lower forceps have their blades set at right-angles to the handles (Fig. 37). Lower root forceps with fine blades are used to extract lower incisors, premolars, and roots, and heavier blades are used to remove canines or large roots. As the mandibular molars have mesial and distal roots, the buccal and

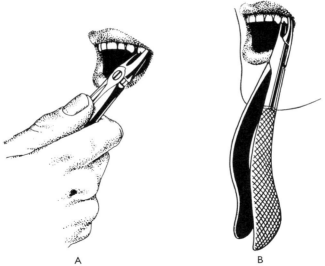

A   B

Fig. 36.—A, The lower lip and incisor teeth prevent the correct application of a pair of straight forceps to a maxillary first premolar. B, The two curves in the Read forceps permit the blades to be applied along the long axis of the tooth.

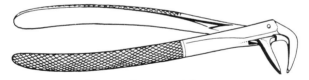

Fig. 37.—Lower root forceps.

lingual blades of lower full molar forceps are similar in design, and the same pair of forceps can be used to extract both right and left mandibular molars.

Dental forceps are designed to grasp the root or root-mass of teeth and *not* the crown. Care must be taken to select a pair of forceps with blades which do not touch the crown when the roots are gripped (*see Fig.* 44, p. 28).

All the factors outlined above govern the choice of the correct pair of forceps to be used for the extraction of a particular tooth. The choice can only be made after careful clinical examination of the tooth, as detailed on page 3.

Extraction with Dental Forceps.—The patient is seated comfortably in the chair with the head-rest adjusted to fit the nape of the neck and support the head (*Fig.* 38). After adjusting the chair to the appropriate height, fitting an apron around the patient's neck, and inspecting the tooth to be extracted, the instruments required for the operation are selected, sterilized, and placed in a sterile dish at the side of the patient, but out of his line of vision. Anaesthesia, either local or general, is then secured (*see* p. 60, Dental Props).

The forceps are then picked up in the operator's *right* hand, which is used to grip and control them. The correct grip is shown in *Fig.* 39 A. The position of the thumb just below the joint of the forceps, and the position of the forceps handles in the palm of the hand, give the operator a firm grip on,

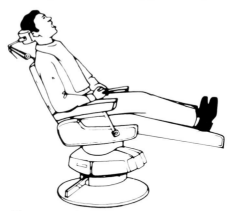

Fig. 38.—Patient seated in the dental chair.

and fine control over, the instrument. The little finger is placed inside the handle and used to control the opening of the forceps blades during their application to the root. When the tooth is gripped the little finger is placed outside the handle (*Fig.* 39 B).

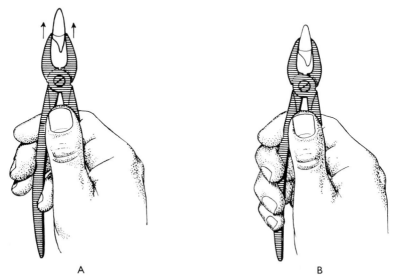

A   B

Fig. 39.—Correct grip of forceps: A, During application of the forceps to the tooth. B, During the extraction of the tooth.

Few dental surgeons are ambidextrous and most of them can only hold and control forceps properly with the right hand. Nevertheless, the left hand has an important role to fulfil during every extraction. The correct use of the *left* hand facilitates extraction greatly. It is used to displace the tongue, cheeks, and lips from the site of extraction to improve visual and mechanical access, and to push the adjacent soft tissues out of harm's way. The left hand supports and fixes the mandible during the removal of mandibular teeth. This is of especial importance when working upon patients under general anaesthesia, because depression of the mandible interferes with the patency of the airway. When extracting teeth under local anaesthesia, support of the

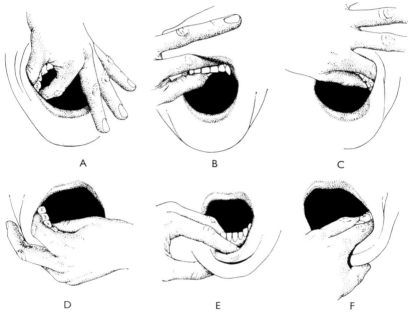

Fig. 40.—Correct use of left hand during the extraction of: A, Right maxillary premolars and molars. B, Maxillary anterior teeth. C, Left maxillary premolars and molars. D, Right mandibular cheek teeth. (N.B. The operator stands behind the patient when extracting these teeth.) E, Mandibular anterior teeth. F, Left mandibular molars and premolars.

mandible lessens the discomfort of the patient, while under either form of anaesthesia support of the mandible facilitates the extraction and prevents dislocation of the temporomandibular joint. The fingers of the left hand grip and support the alveolar bone around the tooth being extracted and transmit information to the operator during the procedure (*Fig.* 40). They are used to compress the socket after the removal of the tooth and to deliver the whole tooth, root, or dislodged fillings from the mouth.

The Application of the Forceps Blades to the Tooth.—After placing the left hand in position and thus obtaining a clear view of the tooth to be extracted, the forceps blades are applied to the buccal and lingual surfaces of the *root* or *root-mass* with their long axes either on or parallel to that of the tooth (*Fig.* 41). The blades are forced through the periodontal membrane between the tooth-root and the investing alveolar bone towards the apex. Firm pressure upon the forceps is used to drive the blades along the surface of the root as far as

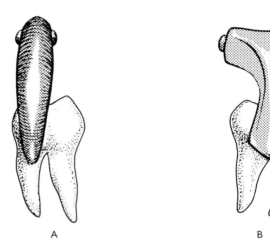

A   B

Fig. 41.—Correct application of forceps blades to a lower molar. A, Lower root forceps. B, Lower molar forceps.

possible. During this procedure the right little finger is used to keep the blades in the periodontal membrane, but when the root or root-mass is gripped this finger should be placed alongside the others outside the forceps handle (*see Fig.* 39 B).

It is a good practice to apply the forceps blade to the less accessible side of the tooth first under direct vision and then apply the other blade. If either the buccal or lingual surface of the tooth is destroyed by cervical caries the appropriate blade should be applied to the carious side first, and the first movement made towards the caries (*Fig.* 42). These measures are designed to ensure that the forceps blade grips the sound tissue of the root thus reducing the risk of fracture of the tooth.

The Displacement of the Tooth from its Socket.—When the blades have been forced as far as possible along the root-surface a firm grip of the root is taken with the forceps, and buccolingual and linguobuccal movements are made in that order. This pressure should be firm, smooth, and controlled, and is applied by the operator moving his trunk from the hips and *not* by moving his elbow. Wrist movements and supination and pronation of the forearm play an essential but lesser part during forceps extraction.

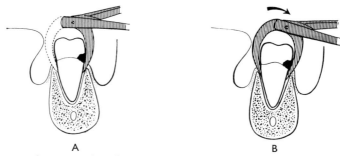

A   B

Fig. 42.—A cross-section of a mandibular molar with cervical caries on its buccal surface. The buccal blade of the forceps is put in position under direct vision (A) and after the application of the lingual blade a buccal movement is made first (B).

Normally, after a few lateral movements, the tooth is felt to loosen and begin to rise out of its socket. When this loosening occurs, rotatory or 'figure-of-eight' movements (*Fig.* 43) will effect delivery of the tooth in a very short period.

The tooth having been delivered and examined to ensure that it is complete (*see Fig.* 54, p. 33 and *Fig.* 94, p. 63), the expanded socket is compressed between the left thumb and forefinger in order to reduce the distortion of both hard and soft supporting tissues. This simple measure materially assists healing.

Sometimes when the tooth is loose in its socket the gum is found to be adhering to its cervical margin. The soft tissue should be carefully dissected from the tooth-neck with either scissors or a scalpel prior to the removal of the tooth. Omission of this step may result in laceration of soft tissues with exposure of the underlying alveolar bone.

If the tooth fails to yield to firm pressure, the forceps must be put down and the cause of the difficulty sought by clinical and radiographic reassessment of the case. In most instances 'transalveolar' removal will be required to complete the extraction (*see* Chapter III).

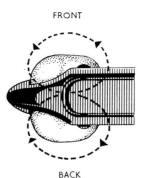

FRONT

BACK

Fig. 43.—Occlusal view of a mandibular molar illustrating 'figure-of-eight' movements.

Rotation of Teeth.—Only the maxillary central incisor and the mandibular second premolar have straight conical roots often enough to permit their detachment from their sockets by a *primary* rotatory movement. If such a tooth is felt to resist rotation it should be moved buccolingually as described above. If rotatory movement is continued in these circumstances, a spiral fracture of the tooth-root may occur. This mishap leaves a root fragment which is difficult to remove, especially when it is retained in the mandibular premolar region.

As stated above, rotatory movements are useful in completing the removal of teeth previously loosened by other means. By the use of this *secondary* rotatory movement, the gross distortion and laceration of the buccal plate and mucosa resulting from excessive lateral movements are avoided.

Common Errors in Forceps Extraction.—Failure to grip the root firmly in the forceps blades during the extraction is a common error. The grip upon the root of the tooth is dependent upon the forceps handles being held firmly together. Failure to do this results in great loss of power and the needless fracture of many teeth.

When there has been no movement in response to the application of moderate force, further attempts to move the root within its socket may result in its fracture and damage to the investing structures, which will delay healing and cause after-pain. The forceps should be put down and the patient

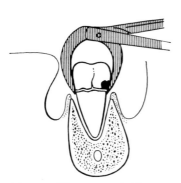

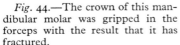

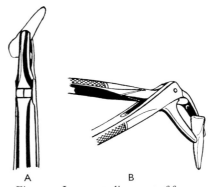

Fig. 44.—The crown of this mandibular molar was gripped in the forceps with the result that it has fractured.

A   B

Fig. 45.—Incorrect alinement of forceps blades to teeth. A, Upper premolar. B, Lower incisor.

allowed to rest while the operator decides whether the 'trans-alveolar' method of extraction should be employed. (*See* Chapter III.)

Another common mistake is to grip the crown in the forceps blades instead of the root or root-mass. This often causes the crown to fracture, especially if it is either carious or heavily restored (*Fig.* 44).

Incorrect alinement of the forceps blades to the long axis of the root is another frequent cause of failure (*Fig.* 45), but perhaps the most common cause is hurry. Forceps extraction is a skilled and delicate procedure, and the good extractor works with an economy of movement and does not yield to the temptation to hurry if he is either uncertain of his anaesthesia or very busy.

Time spent in careful application of forceps blades to the radicular portion of a tooth is never wasted.

If the forceps move upon the root, or if the operator tires, or is in a bad position, it always pays to stop and review the situation. After remedying the underlying error in technique, or having a short rest, the same forceps, or a more suitable pair, are reapplied to the tooth and the extraction completed.

Forceps extraction having been dealt with in general terms, the ways in which this basic technique must be adapted when applied to the extraction of individual teeth must now be considered.

The Extraction of Maxillary Teeth.—

Central incisors have often a conical root and yield to primary rotation (*see* p. 27).

Lateral incisors have slender roots which are often flattened on the mesial and distal surfaces. Choose fine-bladed forceps and get well up the root before applying pressure to the tooth.

Canines have a long, strong, root with a triangular cross-section. Some of the 'canine' forceps have blades which are too wide to give 'two-point contact' if correctly applied well up the root. In many cases these teeth are better dissected out. When multiple extractions are being performed, the chances of fracturing the labial plate while extracting the canine can be reduced by removing this tooth before the lateral incisor and first premolar, as the prior extraction of these teeth weakens the labial plate.

The *maxillary first premolar* has two fine roots which may be both curved and divergent (*Fig.* 46) and fracture occurs readily during extraction. In some cases the long axis of the tooth inclines medially as it goes upwards, its apex being closer to that of the canine than to the apex of the second premolar (*Fig.* 110, p. 82). It is important to note the inclination of the tooth and great care should be taken

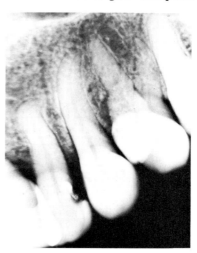

Fig. 46.—A radiograph showing the two slender roots of the maxillary first premolar.

to aline the blades of a fine-bladed forceps along the long axis of the tooth.

It is often taught that this tooth should be pulled out, but, in practice, lateral movements are often required to deliver the tooth with divergent slender roots. If the *predominant lateral movement* is made *towards the buccal side* and radicular fracture occurs, the palatal root is normally delivered whole, leaving the more accessible buccal root to be removed by dissection. If the tooth is pulpless or heavily restored, or if the patient has a history of difficult extractions, an elective trans-alveolar removal is indicated. If the upper first permanent molar is lost the maxillary premolars may drift distally and rotate around their palatal root. This rotation, and the tilting which often accompanies it, must be carefully taken into consideration when the forceps blades are applied to the tooth.

In crowded mouths the *second maxillary premolar* is often instanding. In some cases it is possible to grip the tooth mesiodistally if the forceps are held across the dental arch (*Fig.* 47) and deliver it in this way. If it is not practicable to use this manœuvre the tooth should be removed by dissection.

The roots of the *maxillary first permanent molar* may be widely splayed (*Fig.* 6, p. 4), and if full molar forceps are used care must be taken to make sure that the blades are driven well up the periodontal membrane so as to grip the root-mass. In some cases trans-alveolar extraction with root division is indicated (*see Fig.* 88, p. 56).

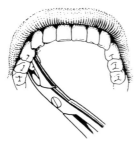

Fig. 47.—The extraction of an in-standing second premolar with forceps.

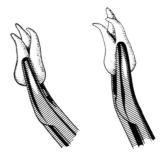

Fig. 48.—Correct positioning of the buccal blade of a pair of Read forceps applied to a right maxillary molar.

If the first molar is lost and the other maxillary molars migrate, they tend to rotate forwards around the palatal root and tilt mesially. In some cases the root-mass of the *maxillary second molar* is set obliquely to the crown, the so-called 'oblique rooted molar'. In both circumstances it may be either difficult or impossible to grip the root-mass with full molar forceps and upper premolar forceps should be used, the buccal blade being carefully placed on either the mesiobuccal or distobuccal root, but never between them (*Fig.* 48).

The long axis of the *maxillary third molar* is such that its crown is usually more posteriorly placed than its roots. This may make difficult the application of forceps, and if the patient's mouth is opened too widely the coronoid process may interfere with access and increase the difficulty. However, if the patient half closes the mouth and a premolar or bayonet forceps is used, usually it is possible to grip the tooth correctly, and buccal pressure delivers it. This buccal movement is facilitated if the patient deviates his mandible towards the side of extraction and thus moves the coronoid process away from the field of operation. In most cases the root has a simple conical form, but occasionally a complicated root pattern will cause the tooth to resist forceps extraction, and in these cases extraction by dissection is indicated (*Fig.* 49).

No attempt should be made to apply forceps to either a semi-erupted maxillary third molar or to the roots of maxillary cheek teeth unless both buccal and lingual surfaces are visible. If pressure is applied in an upward direction the tooth or root may be displaced into the maxillary antrum (*see* Chapter V, p. 74).

The Extraction of Mandibular Teeth.—The *mandibular incisors* have fine roots with flattened sides. They may be very easy to extract but are sometimes very brittle. Fine-bladed forceps should be used.

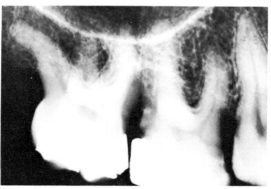

Fig. 49.—This maxillary third molar had five roots and was removed by dissection.

The extraction of the six lower anterior teeth can often be facilitated by loosening them with a straight elevator (*Fig.* 50, *see also* p. 34).

The root of the *mandibular canine* is longer and stouter than that of adjacent teeth. The apex is often inclined distally. A heavier-bladed forceps should be used and special care taken in its application to the tooth.

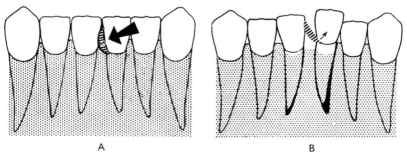

Fig. 50.—Stobie technique. A, A straight elevator is inserted between lower incisors and rotated. B, Both teeth are loosened and the extraction of them with forceps is facilitated.

Mandibular premolars have tapering roots and their apices may be distally inclined. Lower premolar roots are often invested in dense bone and if fractured during extraction usually have to be dissected out. A pair of forceps with blades fine enough to give 'two-point contact' on the root should be carefully applied to the tooth. The first movements should be firm but gentle, and in the case of *second premolars only*, these initial movements may be rotatory. If resistance to this 'primary rotation' is felt it should be abandoned in favour of the more classic lateral movements. If attempts at rotation are continued, a spiral fracture of the root may occur, leaving a root fragment which is difficult to remove.

Lower molars are best extracted with full molar forceps, but many operators do not use these forceps because they find great difficulty in driving the wide blades through the periodontal membrane. Unless care is taken to force the blades well down the periodontal membrane so that the root-mass can be gripped, the crown of the tooth will be crushed in the forceps. For the extraction of a grossly carious tooth many dental surgeons prefer root forceps applied to the root over which most sound crown is present. These teeth are

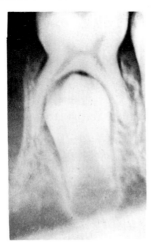 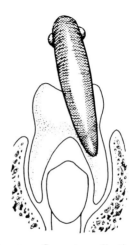

Fig. 51.—Radiograph showing the relationship of deciduous molar roots to the underlying forming premolar.

Fig. 52.—Correct application of forceps blades to a deciduous lower molar.

often loosened by buccolingual pressure and are best delivered by secondary rotation. The extraction of second and third mandibular molars can often be facilitated by the mesial application of an elevator before the application of forceps (*see Fig.* 56, p. 34). This technique must not be used during the removal of lower first permanent molars because with the differing root-patterns of this tooth and the second premolar, the attachments of the latter tooth may be damaged by force transmitted via the interdental septum. The root-pattern of the *mandibular third permanent molar* is so variable that a radiograph should be taken before extraction, even when the tooth is fully erupted. In many instances these teeth are better dissected from their attachments.

The Extraction of Deciduous Teeth.—While the removal of deciduous anterior teeth is usually very easy if the basic technique is employed, the deciduous cheek teeth are sometimes more difficult to extract than their permanent successors. Several factors combine to produce this difficulty. The child's mouth is small and provides limited access, and the forming premolars are enclosed within the roots of their deciduous predecessors and rhus liable to damage when the latter teeth are extracted (*Fig.* 51). Deciduous molars have no root-mass and caries often invades the roots, making it difficult to grip them. Resorption of the roots of teeth of the temporary dentition does not occur in an orderly fashion from the apex towards the crown. Often the side of a root may be resorbed and this may render the retention of root-fragments inevitable.

The technique of extraction of deciduous teeth is basically the same as that used in the removal of permanent teeth. It is especially important when applying forceps to ensure that the blades are fine enough to pass down the periodontal membranes and that they are applied to the roots (*Fig.* 52). If they are just placed on the buccal and lingual sides of the tooth and forced into the tissues the permanent successor may be damaged. A firm lingual movement usually causes the tooth to rise in its socket and it can then be

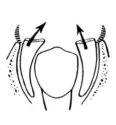

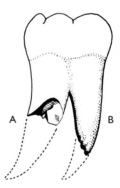

Fig. 53.—The extraction of deciduous molar roots with a Warwick James elevator.

Fig. 54.—A, Fractured root, B, Resorbed root of a permanent mandibular molar.

delivered by being moved buccally and rotated forwards. It is better to leave a small root-fragment of a deciduous tooth to undergo resorption or exfoliation rather than to damage or displace the permanent successor in attempts to locate and remove it. The decision whether to remove such a fragment must be made in each individual case after all the relevant factors have been considered. When removal of it is undertaken the soft tissues must be reflected sufficiently to permit the operator to see the exact relationship of the permanent successor and to enable him to deliver the root-fragment under direct vision.

When applying forceps blades to a root which is carious at gum level, it must be realized that the gum tends to grow over the edges of such roots and the margins of the root must be carefully defined. Deciduous roots which cannot be grasped with forceps should be displaced inwards towards the forming permanent tooth with a Warwick James elevator, using the bony socket wall as the fulcrum (*Fig.* 53). The roots of extracted deciduous teeth should be examined to ensure that they are complete. Fractured root-surfaces are flat and shiny with sharp margins, resorbed roots are ragged and matt with irregular margins (*Fig.* 54, p. 33 and *Fig.* 94, p. 63).

The Use of Elevators.—Elevators are used on the lever and fulcrum principle to force the tooth or root along the line of withdrawal. The *line of withdrawal* is the path along which the tooth or root will move out of its socket with the least application of force to it. This line of least resistance is primarily determined by the root-pattern. The fulcrum used for the elevation of teeth should always be a bony one. The use of an adjacent tooth as a

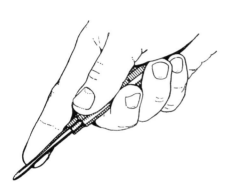
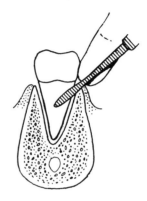

Fig. 55.—Elevator correctly held in the hand.

Fig. 56.—Elevator correctly applied to the mesial surface of a mandibular molar.

fulcrum is only permissible if that tooth is to be extracted at the same visit (*see* p. 31). Elevators may be forced down the periodontal membrane either mesially, buccally, or distally to the tooth being extracted. The elevator should be grasped in the fingers (*Fig.* 55) and forced down the periodontal membrane at an angle of 45° to the long axis of the root (*Fig.* 56). The tip of the index finger rests against the alveolar bone and enables the operator to have complete control over the instrument. The *point of application* of an elevator, that is, the site on the root at which force must be applied to effect delivery, is determined by the line of withdrawal of the tooth or root. If the root is straight and conical it will move upwards and slightly lingually if force is applied to its buccal surface—*buccal application* (*Fig.* 57 A). If the apex of the root points distally the elevator must be applied to the mesial surface of the root—*mesial application*—because the line of withdrawal is upwards and backwards (*Fig.* 57 B). If the apex of the root points mesially a *distal application* is called for to elevate the tooth upwards and forwards out of its socket

(*Fig.* 57 C). When the elevator has been applied to the tooth, the instrument is rotated around its long axis (*Fig.* 58), so that the lower edge of its blade engages upon the cementum covering the root-surface and moves the tooth out of its socket. If a preoperative radiograph is available the line of withdrawal of the root or tooth and the correct point of application for an elevator are readily determined. However, the root-pattern of certain teeth and the shape of some roots are similar so often that many experienced operators use

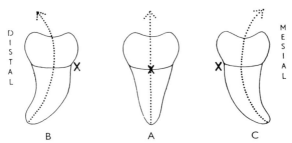

Fig. 57.—Buccal views of three right mandibular molars with differing root patterns to show the lines of withdrawal and points of application of an elevator (×). *See text for explanation.*

elevators to extract them without the benefit of a preoperative radiograph. In these circumstances, if the tooth or root resists elevation when moderate force is applied to it the instrument should be put down and the cause of difficulty sought. The teeth most commonly elevated from their sockets are second and third mandibular molars. The apices of many of these teeth are distally

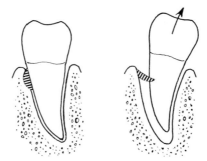

Fig. 58.—Rotation of an elevator around its long axis.

inclined and a mesial application of the elevator is indicated. It is obvious that sometimes the root-pattern will be unfavourable to such elevation, or that in some multi-rooted teeth the lines of withdrawal of the roots might conflict. In these cases mesial application is contra-indicated and should be abandoned. An attempt to drive the roots along a mean path of withdrawal by a buccal application of force or to deliver the tooth with forceps will succeed only if the alveolar bone is sufficiently elastic and yielding and the root-pattern is not too unfavourable. If these measures fail to deliver the tooth, extraction must be performed by the trans-alveolar method (*see* p. 40). An elevator must not be applied mesially to a first mandibular molar in an attempt to loosen it. The mandibular second premolar has a conical root and may be dislocated from its socket by force transmitted through the interdental septum between

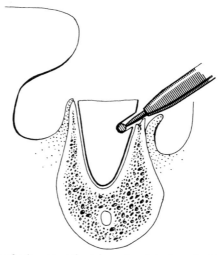

Fig. 59.—The use of a bur to make a buccal point of application for an elevator.

the two teeth. An attempt to apply mesial force to a mandibular third molar is contra-indicated unless the operator is certain that *no* distal bone is present which will prevent the tooth moving along a distal path of withdrawal. In teeth with fused roots it is necessary to provide a buccal point of application for an elevator. This is done by burring into the buccal surface of the root at an angle of 45° to the long axis of the root (*Fig.* 59).

After-care.—When the tooth has been extracted the socket should be inspected and any loose fragment of bone removed or necessary socket toilet performed (*see* p. 48). The socket should then be squeezed in order to reduce any distortion of the supporting tissues, the patient should be allowed to rinse the mouth *once* with a warm bland mouthwash, and then instructed to bite firmly upon a gauze pack until a firm blood-clot is present in the socket. The pack must be arranged so that firm pressure is exerted upon the bleeding socket margins, and the gauze may be enclosed in sterile cellophane to prevent the absorption of blood from the socket (*see Fig.* 105, p. 75).

The dental surgeon's duty to his patient does not end with the placing of a pack or the insertion of the last suture. He must ensure that the patient's postoperative period is as pain-free and uneventful as possible. A suitable analgesic should be prescribed for use as required.

Aspirin.—This is an effective analgesic and also possesses anti-pyretic and anti-inflammatory properties especially when used in high dosage. The efficacy of aspirin is known to be dose-related and when given in single doses of 1000 mg or more the drug has been described as the analgesic of choice. Aspirin remains the most widely used analgesic and either Aspirin tablets B.P. or Aspirin tablets dispersible B.P. are adequate for most purposes as they act rapidly, are inexpensive and are readily available.

However, aspirin may have topical erosive effects on the gastro-intestinal-mucosa and so may cause iron-deficiency anaemia, haematemesis, nausea, or vomiting. Sensitivity reactions which can occur include rashes, swellings, asthma, and even an anaphylactoid reaction in rare instances. Even small

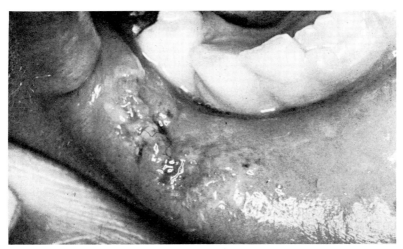

Fig. 60.—An example of ulceration of the lower lip in a child who bit it after receiving an inferior dental injection.

doses of salicylates may prolong the prothrombin time in patients on anti-coagulant therapy. The prescription of aspirin, or mixtures containing aspirin, is contra-indicated in anyone giving a history of sensitivity to the drug or of asthma, in patients afflicted with either peptic ulceration or a haemorrhagic disease, or in those on anticoagulant therapy.

In such patients aspirin-free analgesics must be prescribed.

Paracetamol.—This is a weaker analgesic than aspirin and has no anti-inflammatory action. It does not cause gastric irritation and can be given safely to patients with a history of dyspepsia or peptic ulceration. Paediatric paracetamol elixir is preferable to aspirin in children as it does not cause metabolic acidosis. It is a suitable analgesic for relief of pain in primary herpetic stomatitis.

Overdosage with paracetamol is dangerous as it can cause hepatitic damage which may not become apparent for 4 to 6 days. This complication may occur when the drug is either used on its own or in combination. Paracetamol is often prescribed with dextropropoxyphene (Distalgesic). In overdose this combination has the same danger as paracetamol alone with the added complication of respiratory failure. Even in the recommended dosage paracetamol may in rare instances cause dizziness, sleepiness and gastro-intestinal disturbances.

The pain relief afforded by paracetamol is not dose-related and in view of the danger of hepatotoxicity in overdosage, patients should be warned not to exceed the stated dose.

Codeine Phosphate.—Unlike the drugs previously mentioned this drug belongs to the narcotic group of analgesics. It is used for the control of mild to moderate pain and is frequently combined with non-narcotic analgesics in compound analgesic preparations. Whilst it is claimed to be more effective when used in such formulations, its analgesic action is said by many authorities to be low. Constipation may complicate its repeated use and patients should be counselled against the ingestion of large amounts of the drug.

Popular Analgesic Preparations containing Aspirin.—

1. Aspirin tablets B.P., each tablet containing Aspirin 300 mg. Adult dose: 1–3 tablets every 4–6 hours when necessary. Maximum dose: gr. 4 daily.

2. Aspirin tablets dispersible B.P., same as Aspirin tablets B.P., but in an effervescent base.

3. Paynocil, a proprietary product, each tablet containing Aspirin 600 mg. (gr. 10) and Amino acetic acid 300 mg. (gr. 5). Adult dose: 1 or 2 tablets 4-hourly to control pain.

4. Aspirin and Codeine tablet dispersible B.P., each tablet containing Aspirin 400 mg. and Codeine phosphate 8 mg. in an effervescent base. Adult dose: 1–2 tablets 4-hourly when necessary.

5. Aspirin, Paracetamol and Codeine tablets D.P.F., each tablet containing Aspirin 250 mg., Paracetamol 250 mg. and Codeine phosphate 6–8 mg. Adult dose: 1–2 tablets 4-hourly when necessary. Maximum dose: 8 tablets daily.

Popular Aspirin-free Analgesic Preparations.—

1. Paracetamol tablets B.P., each tablet containing Paracetamol 500 mg. Adult dose: 1–2 tablets every 4–6 hours when necessary. Maximum dose: 8 tablets daily.

2. Paracetamol Elixir, Paediatric B.P., Paracetamol 120 mg. in 5 ml. Not to be diluted. Dosage: Child up to 1 year 60–120 mg.; 1–5 years 120–240 mg.; 6–12 years 240–480 mg. These doses may be repeated every 4–6 hours when necessary.

3. Distalgesic, a proprietary product, each tablet containing Dextropropoxyphene hydrochloride 32·5 mg. and Paracetamol 325 mg. Adult dose: 2 tablets 3–4 times a day when necessary. Maximum dose: 10 tablets daily.

4. Codeine phosphate tablets B.P., each tablet containing Codeine phosphate 30 mg. Adult dose: 10–60 mg. (gr. 1/6–1) every 4 hours when necessary. Maximum dose: 200 mg. daily.

5. Codeine and Paracetamol tablets dispersible B.P.C., each tablet containing Codeine phosphate 8 mg. and Paracetamol 500 mg. in an effervescent

base. Adult dose: 1–2 tablets every 4–6 hours when necessary. Maximum dose: 8 tablets daily.

These tablets have been found to be of value only in the control of mild pain and two other aspirin-free proprietary preparations are usually employed when a patient is expected to have more severe pain.

The first of these is Mefenamic acid (Ponstan) which is an effective analgesic with properties similar to those of aspirin. The indications for and contra indications to its use are also similar to those of aspirin. It has been found to be effective in an adult dosage of 2 kapseals (500 mg.) orally followed by 1 kapseal (250 mg.) every 6 hours. It is wise to prescribe it in quantities suitable for a few days use only. This drug should be used with caution in patients with renal impairment or peptic ulceration, and its use should be discontinued if diarrhoea or skin rashes occur, or there is depression of the white cell count. It should not be prescribed for either epileptic or pregnant patients.

The other preparation is Diflunisal (Dolobid), a non-steroidal anti-inflammatory analgesic, with a relatively long duration of action. It has peripheral analgesic, anti-inflammatory and weak antipyretic effects, and inhibits synthesis of prostaglandins and platelet aggregation less than aspirin. The recommended adult dose is 1000 mg., followed by 500 mg. twice a day. In this dosage the drug appears to be more effective than aspirin and its effects last from 8 to 12 hours. It causes less gastric irritation than aspirin but should be used with caution, if at all, in pregnant women. Other than in hospital practice, there is seldom a need for a dental surgeon to use addictive drugs which are subject to legal control.

The patient should be instructed to avoid vigorous mouthwashing, violent exercise, stimulants, or very hot food or drink for the rest of the day to minimize the risk of post-extraction haemorrhage. Before the patient is discharged he should be shown how to place either a gauze pressure pack or a clean folded handkerchief upon the socket and bite upon it firmly in order to arrest any haemorrhage which might occur.

The extraction wound should be cleansed by rinsing the mouth with warm saline immediately before going to bed on the day of operation. Healing may be aided by the use of hot saline mouth-baths frequently during the following two or three days. The solution is prepared by dissolving half a teaspoonful of salt in a tumbler of hot, but not scalding, water. Copious amounts should be taken into the mouth as frequently as is practicable and held over the site of extraction for as long as is possible. The use of mouth-baths is particularly helpful when undertaken immediately after meals and before going to bed.

Following the use of local anaesthesia the lips, tongue, or cheeks may remain numb for two or three hours during which they may be damaged by biting (Fig. 60). The patient should be warned of this danger and instructed to return for consultation should anything untoward complicate the healing period.

Whenever it is practicable to do so verbal post-extraction instructions should be supplemented by giving the patient either a printed or written copy of the instructions.

CHAPTER III

TRANS-ALVEOLAR EXTRACTION

THIS method of extraction comprises the dissection of a tooth or root from its bony attachments. It is often called the 'open' or 'surgical' method. As all extractions, however performed, are surgical procedures, a better and more accurate name is 'trans-alveolar' extraction, and the method should be used when any of the following indications are present:—

1. Any tooth which resists attempts at intra-alveolar extraction when moderate force is applied.

2. Retained roots which cannot be either grasped with forceps or delivered with an elevator, especially those in relationship to the maxillary antrum.

3. A history of difficult or attempted extractions.

4. Any heavily restored tooth, especially when root filled or pulpless.

5. Hypercementosed and ankylosed teeth.

6. Geminated and dilacerated teeth.

7. Teeth shown radiographically to have complicated root patterns, or roots with unfavourable or conflicting lines of withdrawal.

8. When it is desired to insert a denture either immediately or soon after extraction. The method facilitates any judicious trimming of the alveolar bone which may be required to enable the prosthesis to be inserted.

Having decided to employ the *trans-alveolar* method to remove a tooth or root, the type of anaesthesia to be used (*see* p. 10) should be decided, and an overall plan to overcome the difficulties and either avoid or deal with any possible complications should be formulated. Important components of such a plan are the design of the mucoperiosteal flap, the method to be used to deliver the tooth or roots from the socket, and the bone removal required to facilitate this.

Mucoperiosteal Flaps.—These are raised to render the operative site clearly visible and accessible and their design should ensure that they provide adequate visual and mechanical access. The base of such a flap should be broader than its free end and must contain an unimpaired blood-supply. Healing by first intention will not occur if the suture lines are placed over blood-clot, which is a perfect culture medium for the micro-organisms which cause breakdown of wounds. Attempts to promote healing should be made by accurately apposing the soft tissues without tension at the end of the operation, and so designing the incisions that the suture lines are supported by bone (*Figs.* 61, 62). Prosthetic difficulties should not be produced as a result of obliteration of the buccal sulcus during the raising of flaps (*see* p. 43).

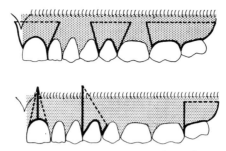

Fig. 61.—Maxillary mucoperiosteal flaps. *Top*: Good flaps. *Bottom*: Bad flaps.

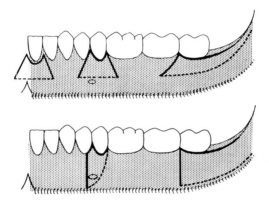

Fig. 62.—Mandibular mucoperiosteal flaps. *Top*: Good flaps. *Bottom*: Bad flaps.

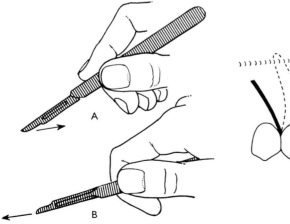

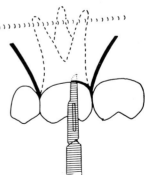

Fig. 63.—A, Correct and B, Incorrect use of a scalpel.

Fig. 64.—Vertical incision of the cervical margin of a standing tooth.

The *incision* should be made with firm pressure upon a sharp scalpel through both the mucous and periosteal layers of the gingiva down to the bone. The scalpel should be used as a pen and not as a plough (*Fig.* 63), and the soft tissues should be cut at right-angles to the surface of the underlying bone. Incisions of adequate length should be made in one operation, as extensions and 'second cuts' often leave ragged flap margins and delay healing.

When the gingival margin of a standing tooth is involved in the flap it should be incised vertically, as shown in *Fig.* 64, before any attempt is made to raise the flap with the periosteal elevator. Sometimes it is necessary to reflect the mucoperiosteum from adjacent teeth which are to be retained (e.g., from the maxillary second molar during the removal of semi-erupted maxillary

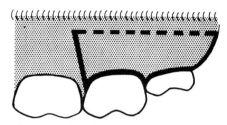 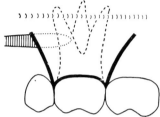

Fig. 65.—Standard incision for the removal of a maxillary third molar.

Fig. 66.—Periosteal elevator inserted to reflect mucoperiosteal flap.

third molars (*Fig.* 65)). If clean incisions are made and the tissues are accurately replaced, the depth of the gingival pocket of the retained tooth will be clinically unaltered when healing is complete.

The mucoperiosteal flap is elevated from the bone by inserting the sharp end of a periosteal elevator under the anterior edge of the flap a few millimetres away from the gingival margin (*Fig.* 66). It is easier to find the correct tissue plane at this site than elsewhere. Compact bone will be exposed if the incision has been made through both layers of the gingiva. If the incision is not deep enough, the flap will resist elevation and the bone will be covered with strands of fibrous periosteum, which should be divided with the scalpel before further attempts are made to raise the flap. If the incision is of inadequate depth the mucous and periosteal layers of the mucoperiosteum are separated when elevation of the flap is attempted, rendering accurate replacement of the soft tissues at the end of the operation impossible, and consequently healing is delayed.

The Advantages of Large Flaps.—It is always good practice to create large flaps in the horizontal plane rather than small ones. A flap which is long in its anteroposterior dimension provides adequate visual and mechanical access without the necessity of stretching or pulling the soft tissues. Healing by first intention is promoted because the flap has a good blood-supply, does not fall into the bony defects created during the operation, and the suture lines lie upon a firm bony base and not over blood-clot.

There are several disadvantages of overextending flaps in a vertical direction. If the flap is extended to the reflection of the mucous membrane, the alveolar attachment of the buccinator muscle is detached from the bone and a small haematoma results. This causes an increase in postoperative extraoral swelling, and organization of the blood-clot, with resultant fibrosis, may cause a loss of depth in the buccal sulcus. The nerve and vessels passing through the mental foramen may be damaged during the elevation of mucoperiosteal flaps in the mandibular premolar region, especially if soft-tissue dissection extends below the level of the reflection of the mucous membrane.

Flap elevation may be complicated by fibrosis resulting from chronic inflammation or scarring, due to ill-fitting dentures. It is often more difficult

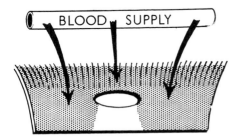

Fig. 67.—A 'button-holed' flap. The blood-supply of the non-shaded area is prejudiced by the artefact.

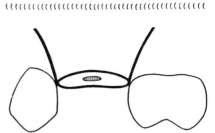

Fig. 68.—The excision of a sinus during the outlining of a flap.

to raise a flap in an edentulous area than in an area where teeth are standing. This is particularly so if the edentulous mucoperiosteum is either very thick or thin and atrophic, as in the post-menopausal period. Holing the flap during its elevation prejudices the blood-supply of the tissue distal to the 'button-hole' (*Fig.* 67). Sinuses are surrounded by chronically inflamed granulation and fibrous tissue, and this has the effect of 'button-holing' any flap which they traverse. It is sometimes possible to incorporate a sinus into the incision line to avoid the flap being 'button-holed' by the sinus and thus eliminate the chronically inflamed tissue (*Fig.* 68).

Bone Removal.—The surface of the alveolar bone investing the tooth or roots to be extracted is exposed when the mucoperiosteal flap is raised, and in most cases it will be necessary to remove some of this bone. Alveolar bone must not be sacrificed unnecessarily and removal of it must be limited to what is required to achieve certain objectives. Before the delivery of the tooth or root, bone should only be excised to expose either of these, to provide a point of application for an elevator or forceps, and to create a space into which the tooth or root may be displaced. After the tooth or root has been delivered all sharp edges and bony projections should be removed. In some cases further excision of bone may be indicated, either to reduce the size of the blood-clot by reducing the size of the socket, or to eliminate an obstacle to postoperative prosthetic success.

Bone is usually removed either with a dental bur or by the use of a chisel or gouge with hand or mallet pressure. Usually bone removal by the correct use of a sharp chisel is quicker and cleaner than removal by bur, which, however, is more suitable for the removal of dense mandibular bone under local anaesthesia. Most dental surgeons handle a bur more frequently and more efficiently than a chisel. Rongeur forceps (*Fig.* 69) are valuable instruments for trimming bone edges after extraction of the tooth or root. The operator must choose his method of bone removal according to his own particular skills and the facilities available to him. Maxillary buccal and labial plate can be removed with a chisel, as shown in *Fig.* 70, except when the bone is very sclerotic or the root is fractured below the level of the bony socket margin, when recourse to a bur is preferable. Most dental surgeons find that mandibular bone is best removed with a bur in a straight handpiece.

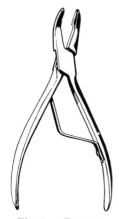

Fig. 69.—Rongeur forceps.

Removal of Bone by Dental Burs.—For this purpose, round or 'rose-head' burs cut more efficiently, do not clog as readily, and are easier to control than flat fissure types, which are more suited to remove bone alongside the periodontal membrane ('guttering'), as they do not cut into the tooth substance so readily. The excellent Ash surgical burs (Toller's pattern) cut even the most dense mandibular bone quickly and efficiently.

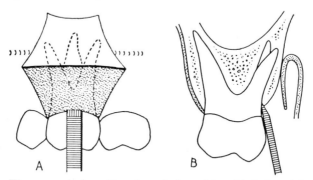

Fig. 70.—The removal of maxillary buccal plate with a chisel viewed from A, the side, and B, the front.

The mucoperiosteal flap should be held away from the site on which the bur is to be used with a flat-bladed retractor. Large flaps facilitate this procedure. By this means, the common 'accident' of the bur burying itself in the soft tissues is prevented.

The bur must never be allowed to overheat during bone removal, and either constant or at least frequent irrigations with sterile normal saline should be used to prevent this, and also to remove debris and prevent the bur from clogging.

Bone may be removed with burs, either by simply cutting it away, using a size No. 8 or 10 round or flat fissure pattern, or by the use of the 'postage-stamp' method. In this technique a row of small holes is made with a small bur (e.g., a size No. 3 round), and then joined together with either bur or chisel cuts (*Fig.* 71). When lower premolar roots are being dissected out, bone removal should be maximal medial to the first premolar and distal to the second premolar. This simple procedure minimizes the risk of damage to the nerve and vessels traversing the mental foramen.

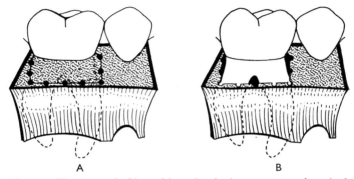

Fig. 71.—The removal of buccal bone by the 'postage-stamp' method.

Dislocation of the tooth or root from its socket should be accomplished by the use of either the dental forceps, if a firm grip of the root or root-mass can be obtained, or by the use of elevators (*see* p. 34).

Tooth Division.—It is obvious that the lines of withdrawal of different roots of some multi-rooted teeth will conflict (*Fig.* 72), and in these cases either forceps removal or a buccal application of an elevator will deliver the tooth if the alveolar bone is sufficiently elastic and yielding and the roots are not too widely splayed. If these measures do not succeed, the root-mass must be divided and the separated roots removed along their individual paths of withdrawal.

The root-mass should be divided with either Ash surgical or standard dental burs (round and fissure patterns). This technique allows the cut to be positioned very accurately and creates a space between the separated roots which aids their removal. Before this, however, the operator must provide points of application to facilitate delivery of the roots. It is folly to divide a tooth leaving the roots deeply embedded in bone.

When the root mass of a lower molar is to be divided, the bifurcation should be exposed and the roots separated from below upwards with a bur (*Fig.* 73). When using this method the operator knows when the roots are completely divided, whereas it is often difficult to be certain if he cuts down towards the bifurcation from above. The separated roots are then delivered with small elevators using the points of application dictated by their individual lines of withdrawal.

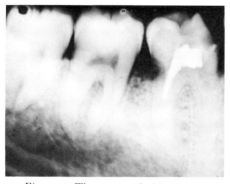

Fig. 72.—The roots of this pulpless mandibular first molar have conflicting lines of withdrawal, and are set in dense sclerotic bone.

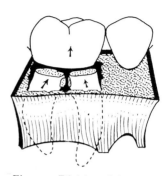

Fig. 73.—Division of the roots of a mandibular first molar.

Bur division of teeth is time-consuming and the experienced oral surgeon may prefer to use an osteotome or a chisel. The student is warned, however, that this simple-looking procedure is not so easy as it might at first appear.

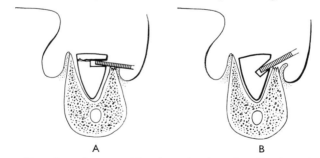

A   B

Fig. 74.—Use of an elevator with a buccal point of application. A, Incorrect angulation of notch. B, Correct angulation of notch.

Tooth-splitting forceps are mentioned only to condemn them, as the operator has no control over the line of split and comminution of the tooth often complicates their use.

When applying buccal force it is necessary to engage the elevator in a notch on the side of the root-mass. In lower molars the bifurcation often suffices, but if no natural notch is present on the root one should be created with a round bur directed at an angle of 45° to the vertical long axis of the root (see Fig. 74 and Fig. 59, p. 36).

The elevators illustrated in *Fig.* 75 are those in everyday use by the author. The Winter 'exolevers' with the corkscrew-type handles (*Fig.* 76) are very powerful and great force (sufficient to fracture the mandible) may be applied with them if they are held as shown in *Fig.* 76 A. Excessive force is never necessary if the principles outlined above are followed, and the correct grip on the 'exolevers' is shown in *Fig.* 76 B. If a tooth or root resists elevation the elevator should be discarded and the cause (e.g., tooth or bone interfering with the line of withdrawal) sought and remedied.

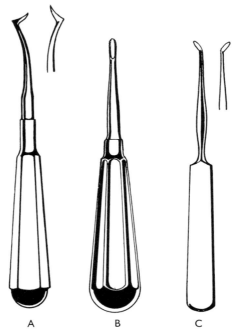

A   B   C

Fig. 75.—Elevators. A, Cryer. B, Lindo Levien. C, Warwick James.

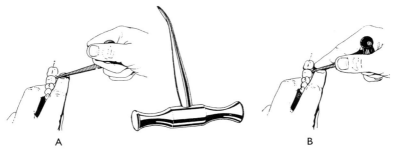

A   B

Fig. 76.—Winter's pattern elevator ('exolever') (*inset*). A, Showing incorrect use of this instrument and B, the correct use.

Socket Toilet.—Removal of the tooth does not complete the operation, and the progress of healing and the amount of after-pain are greatly influenced by the care with which postoperative socket toilet is performed.

Unwanted bony prominences should be removed with either rongeur forceps, chisels, or burs, and sharp edges smoothed with either bone files or plain and cross-cut 'vulcanite' burs (*Fig.* 77). The bone files are toothed to cut only in one direction and are not so useful in dental surgery as the 'vulcanite' burs which cut quickly and cleanly and are easy to use anywhere in the mouth. Rongeur forceps should be used as 'bone scissors' and not with a twisting action.

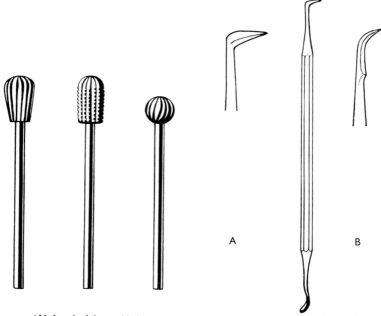

Fig. 77.—'Vulcanite' burs (Ash's acrylic trimmers. Patterns 8, 6, 20R).

Fig. 78.—The Mitchell trimmer (A) and the Cumine scaler (B) differ only in the shape of one end. They are most useful instruments for curettage.

Judicious bone removal will speed healing by reducing the amount of bone to be resorbed and remodelled and the volume of blood-clot which fills the socket.

When any necessary bone removal is complete and the bone edges are smooth, the wound should be irrigated with warm normal saline and all bone debris and infected granulation tissue removed by the use of either a Mitchell trimmer or a Cumine scaler (*Fig.* 78). The mucoperiosteal flap should then be replaced and a decision made as to whether sutures are needed.

Suturing.—Every suture is a foreign body and they should only be inserted into the tissues if there is a positive indication for their use. During the operation a suture may be inserted to retract a mucoperiosteal flap from the field of operation. At the end of an oral surgical operation sutures are inserted

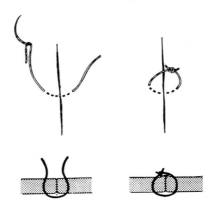

Fig. 79.—Simple interrupted suture.

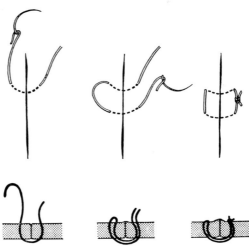

Fig. 80.—Interrupted horizontal mattress suture.

either to hold the cut edges of the soft tissues together to promote healing by first intention, to appose loosely the soft tissues to minimize wound contamination with food debris, or to arrest haemorrhage. If the flap lies snugly in position and bleeding is controlled there is no need for suturing. Where the insertion of sutures is indicated sterile black silk (gauge 000) is the material of choice and either a simple interrupted suture (*Fig.* 79) or an interrupted horizontal mattress suture (*Fig.* 80) should be inserted. Mattress sutures are more trouble to insert, but do not cut out of friable tissues so readily and may also be used to evert flap margins when required. A Lane's No. 3 (22-mm.) cutting needle is widely used in dentistry. The silk can be held in the needle, without a knot, if it is threaded through the eye twice.

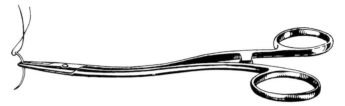

Fig. 81.—Needle held in needle-holders.

Technique of Suturing.—The needle is grasped in needle-holders as shown in *Fig.* 81; it must never be held by the eye or the point. The area to be sutured is dried with either a sucker or a swab so that the cut edges are clearly

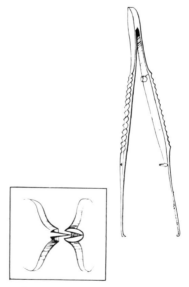

Fig. 82.—Toothed dissecting tweezers. Inset shows a magnified view of the 'mouse-toothed' beaks.

visible. The needle is usually passed through the more mobile flap first, the curve of the needle being used to rotate it through the tissues. Toothed dissecting tweezers (*Fig.* 82) are used to grip the flap and steady it, and the needle should be inserted close to the tips of the beaks (*Fig.* 83) and

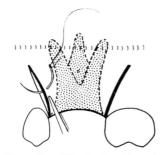

Fig. 83.—Toothed dissecting tweezers hold the flap during the insertion of a suture.

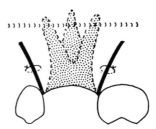

Fig. 84.—Well-placed sutures.

at least 3 mm ($\frac{1}{8}$ in.) from any edge. The suture should be placed closer to the free end of the flap than its base. This controls the most mobile part of the flap and ensures that the suture is in good holding tissue—the mucoperiosteum (*Fig.* 84)—and not in friable mucous membrane. The needle should be passed through one side at a time (*Fig.* 85 A), and in a

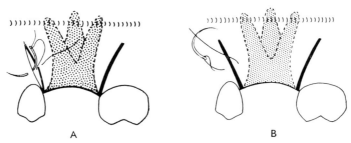

A   B

Fig. 85.—A, Suture needle passing through the attached mucoperiosteum. B, Before the knot is tied tension is exerted on the silk to confirm that the tissues are correctly apposed.

definite arc so that it will emerge in such a position that it may be grasped easily. Slightly freeing the attached mucoperiosteum from the bone enables the needle to be passed through it more readily with less risk of cutting out. It also facilitates the accurate localization of the second puncture. When the suture has been inserted through both flaps the position of the flap should be checked when tension is exerted on the suture (*Fig.* 85 B). If the suture is correctly positioned it should be tied; if not, it should be removed and a new suture inserted. Sutures should always be tied loosely to allow for any slight swelling of the soft tissues and the knots should lie to one side of the incision line (*see Fig.* 84). The knot can be tied either with the fingers or with instruments (*Fig.* 86), and if placed in the buccal or labial sulcus will not worry the tongue.

The first suture determines the success of the suturing. It must be correctly sited if the soft tissues are to be apposed without tension. Full use should be made of landmarks in positioning it, and if it is not correct it should be removed and replaced before further sutures are inserted. When placing

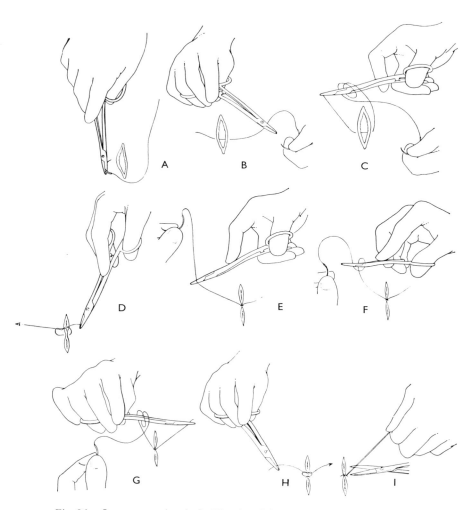

Fig. 86.—Instrument tie. A, B, The tip of the needle-holder is pointed at the needle and passed *over* the silk twice. C, D, The tip of the short end of the silk is grasped and drawn through the loops. E, F, The needle-holders are pointed towards the needle once again and passed *under* the silk once or twice. G, The tip of the short end is then grasped and pulled through the loops, thus completing the knot. H, The loose ends are used to draw the knot to one side of the suture line, and I, then cut with scissors.

a suture in the mandibular lingual mucoperiosteum, the needle should always be passed in a linguobuccal direction away from the tongue. The use of a tongue retractor facilitates this procedure. The needle tip must never be driven into the bone or it will break.

After-care.—The routine for after-care described on page 36 is carried out and arrangements made for a postoperative check-up 48 hours after the extraction. The patient is instructed to return immediately should anything untoward occur before this appointment. It is sound practice to notify the patient's general medical practitioner of every surgical procedure performed upon his patient, however minor it may be.

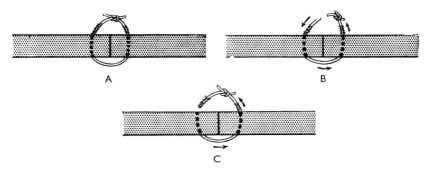

Fig. 87.—A, An intra-oral silk suture is loose and impregnated with food detritus at the end of a week. If it is cut just below the knot, as in B, the wound is contaminated as infected silk is pulled through the tissues. C, This complication is avoided if the silk is cut just as it enters the tissues.

The Removal of Sutures.—The sutures should usually remain in situ for up to 7 days. They loosen in the tissues (*Fig.* 87 A) and should be removed by grasping the knot and cutting the silk where it enters the tissues (*Fig.* 87 C). The suture can then be withdrawn. If the suture is cut at a distance from the point of entry into the tissues (*Fig.* 87 B) contaminated suture material will be dragged through the healing wound, thus infecting it. Sutures inserted to control haemorrhage can be removed 48 hours postoperatively, while sutures used to repair an oro-antral communication are left in situ for at least 10 days unless they become infected.

Summary

The use of a systematic approach enables the dentist to choose the correct method of tooth removal, overcome difficulties, and either completely avoid or effectively deal with possible complications. The steps may be summarized as follows:

1. *Diagnosis and Treatment Planning.*—Careful history taking and clinical examination supplemented by special methods of examination when indicated enable potential difficulties to be assessed, possible complications to be considered, and the correct choice of extraction technique to be made.

2. *Decisions to be taken Prior to Surgery.*—

a. Out-patient or in-patient procedure? Determined by:—

i. General medical condition of patient.

ii. Probable duration of operation.

iii. Type of anaesthesia indicated.

b. Any special arrangements required?

i. Instructions to patient (e.g., not to drive motor vehicle, whether to take meals, probable length of incapacity, whether he should be accompanied, etc.).

ii. ? Desirability of premedication.

iii. ? Any indication for antibiotic cover.

iv. ? Any need for other forms of medical treatment (e.g., anticonvulsants, insulin, anticoagulant or steroid therapy, etc.).

3. *At Operation.*—

a. Ensure that all instruments which may be needed are available and sterilized. (Requirements may be compiled by thinking of each stage of the procedure and listing the instruments needed to perform it.)

b. Lay out instruments in a regular order either in a sterile tray or on a dry disinfected trolley top covered with sterile towels.

c. When single-ended instruments are used, only the handles should be touched.

d. After use instruments should be returned to their former place on the trolley top or in the tray. Soiled swabs should be placed in a separate receptacle.

e. Other requirements: good light, skilled assistance, radiographs of operation site, effective anaesthesia, and an operation plan designed to cope with difficulties and avoid complications.

4. *Postoperative.*—

a. Prescribe analgesics as required.

b. Give clear instructions regarding:—

i. Oral hygiene including the use of hot saline mouth baths.

ii. Haemorrhage, after-pain, and postoperative swelling.

iii. Indications for emergency treatment and arrangements available for it.

c. Make a follow-up appointment.

CHAPTER IV

EXTRACTION TECHNIQUE UNDER GENERAL ANAESTHESIA IN THE DENTAL CHAIR

WHEN a tooth is to be extracted, a decision must be taken whether to employ either local or general anaesthesia. The factors governing the choice of anaesthesia are discussed on page 10, and no general anaesthetic should be administered unless a careful history has been taken and any necessary clinical examination performed. To induce and maintain general anaesthesia, to preserve the airway, and to assist the operator by supporting the mandible while positioning the patient's head to facilitate extraction is a full-time job, if anoxia and other complications are to be avoided. *The dental surgeon should never act as both operator and anaesthetist at the same time.*

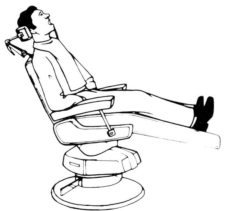

Fig. 90.—Position of the patient in the dental chair during the extraction of a tooth under general anaesthesia.

Preparation for Anaesthesia.—A patient attending a dental surgeon for an extraction under general anaesthesia should be accompanied by a responsible adult and should *not* be in charge of a motor vehicle. He should have had nothing to eat or drink for the 6 hours preceding the operation. After the bladder has been emptied and all tight clothing (collars, belts, etc.) loosened, the patient is seated comfortably in the dental chair with the head slightly extended and the mandible horizontal and parallel to the floor when the mouth is open (*Fig.* 90). It is sound practice always to have a female attendant present when general anaesthetics are administered to female patients. Male patients should be asked to put their hands in their trouser pockets, and female patients are requested to place their hands in their laps with the fingers linked. These simple measures prevent the patient waving his arms about during induction. The chair should have no footpiece and the patient's legs should not be crossed but placed in the position shown in *Fig.* 90. A waterproof apron should be placed around the patient's neck to protect his clothing.

Hearing is the last sense to be lost under general anaesthesia, and the first to be regained as consciousness returns. It is, therefore, of great importance that everyone present, except the anaesthetist, should remain absolutely quiet during the induction and recovery phases. Two common causes of a stormy induction are the ringing of a telephone and the clinking of instruments during the second or 'excitement' stage of anaesthesia. If there is a telephone in the surgery when an anaesthetic is to be administered the receiver should be taken off the hook before induction and replaced after recovery. Instrument trays should be lined with rubber sheeting and have rubber tubing around the edges to reduce the metallic clinking made as the operator selects the instruments required for the extraction.

Preoperative Considerations.—The operator must remember that once the patient is unconscious his co-operation is lost, and so it is important to check every detail before the induction, in addition to taking certain other precautions when extracting teeth under these circumstances.

The identity of the patient and the teeth to be extracted are confirmed. After this any dentures, removable bridgework, or orthodontic appliances are removed and the mouth carefully examined. Whenever possible, the teeth should have been scaled before the extraction. The presence of painful teeth, roots, loose teeth, and large restorations, fixed bridges, and crowns are noted and brought to the attention of the anaesthetist. Any fractured or chipped incisors should be noted, the patient told about them and an entry made in the patient's records preoperatively. After confirming the teeth to be extracted the operator must decide how much to do on this occasion, how he will perform the extractions, and which instruments he will require. The amount of surgery performed under a general anaesthetic in the dental chair is governed by many factors such as any difficulties encountered in performing the extractions and in maintaining anaesthesia. Modern anaesthesia has reached a stage of development where safety and good operating conditions are assured if an anaesthetist skilled in these techniques is employed. It must be remembered, however, that the longer the anaesthetic the more risk there is of anoxia and the inhalation of blood, saliva, pus, or dental fragments. Most authorities feel that inhalational general anaesthesia in the dental chair should not be maintained for longer than 5 to 10 minutes, although some very experienced dental anaesthetists can maintain anaesthesia for 15 to 20 minutes. The operator should never start an operation unless he can finish it, and so he should pay great attention to estimating the time it will take. One difficult extraction may be more time-consuming than ten easy extractions, and multi-rooted teeth are usually more difficult to extract than single-rooted teeth. When average extractions are being performed it is wise to limit the extractions to the equivalent of twelve roots on one occasion e.g., four upper molars or twelve anterior teeth. The operator should attempt to streamline his technique to minimize instrument changes and changes of side. *All* the instruments which might be needed should be selected and arranged in order of use. Care must be taken to ensure that any recently sterilized instruments are cooled before use.

Dental Props.—A dental prop should then be selected and inserted between the jaws on the side opposite to the operative site. A small prop placed well back provides much more room for the operator than a large prop placed more anteriorly, without opening the jaws more widely (*Fig.* 91). A chain attached to the prop is left hanging out of the mouth and should be covered with rubber tubing to avoid chafing the lips. Access will be further impeded when

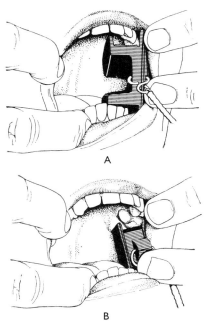

Fig. 91.—Dental props in position between the teeth. A, A large prop placed too far anteriorly limits the amount of intra-oral space available to the operator. B, A small prop placed at the back of the mouth opens the jaws just as widely and provides more space.

the mouth is packed under anaesthesia. After the insertion of the prop the patient should be instructed to relax, close his eyes, and listen to the anaesthetist, who then induces anaesthesia.

Mouth Gags.—These instruments are used for patients who either cannot, or will not, tolerate a prop (e.g., small children) or for those in whom the prop has slipped or been spat out during the induction. The operator may wish to extract right and left teeth at the same sitting, and it is a common practice to insert a gag on the side on which extractions have been performed and remove the prop. Then, after checking that the mouth pack is still occluding the oropharynx, the extractions are completed while the mouth is held open by the gag. Mouth gags are instruments of force and unless great care is taken in their use teeth may be either damaged or displaced, fillings dislodged, and soft tissues bruised. The blades of the gag should be covered with rubber, and the operator should guide their insertion and ensure that they are placed upon teeth or mucoperiosteum which will withstand pressure. The anaesthetist should open them gently and support the gag during the extraction (*Fig.* 92). The gag should never be used to overcome trismus because the natural

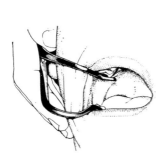

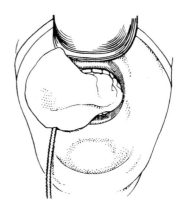

Fig. 92.—A mouth gag in use to keep   Fig. 93.—A mouth pack in position.
         the mouth open.

defensive barriers around an area of infection may easily be broken down by such a procedure. Whenever possible it is best to avoid the use of gags altogether, and usually the skilled dental anaesthetist can relax his patient sufficiently to allow props to be inserted instead of gags.

Mouth Packs.—When the induction is complete and the patient anaesthetized the mouth pack is inserted (*Fig.* 93). It should occlude the oropharynx and is used to prevent the inhalation of foreign bodies, such as teeth, roots, fillings, or pieces of calculus, into the respiratory tract. A piece of Gamgee tissue, 23 cm. (9 in.) long and 6 cm. (2½ in.) wide, is a popular pack, which absorbs any blood, saliva, or pus present at the back of the mouth, thus preventing the risk of inhalation or of laryngeal spasm. The tongue should be displaced to the opposite side when the pack is inserted, and should not be pushed backwards into such a position that the airway is occluded. The tail of the pack should be left protruding from the patient's mouth. It is possible to insert this type of pack quickly and position it correctly by using the following technique. The dentist grasps the pack in his right hand with the tip of his extended index finger situated a little below the longitudinal midline of the pack and about 4 cm. (1½ in.) from its free end. The tip of the index finger is then used to insert the pack into the appropriate lingual sulcus between the side of the tongue and the lingual surface of the mandible. The free end of the pack passes around the distal surface of the last standing tooth and into the buccal sulcus, thus effectively separating the site of operation from the pharynx. Many anaesthetists prefer to insert the mouth pack, but the operator must ensure that the oropharynx is completely occluded before starting the operation. *Under no circumstances should he work without a mouth pack.*

Modification of Extraction Technique.—The correct use of the left hand is of especial importance when extracting teeth under general anaesthesia (*see* p. 25), for if the mandible is depressed unduly the airway will become obstructed and the temporomandibular joint may be dislocated. Teeth should be extracted in a systematic fashion. Very loose and painful teeth are extracted first. Roots are extracted before whole teeth, lower teeth before uppers, and posterior teeth before anterior teeth, so that vision is not obstructed by bleeding from the sockets of teeth already extracted. All the extractions on one side should be completed before extractions are started on the other side.

Care must be taken *not* to trap soft tissues, especially the floor of the mouth, in the blades of the forceps, and to avoid crushing the lower lip between the handles of upper forceps and the lower teeth.

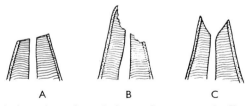

Fig. 94.—Vertical sections through incomplete roots. A, Fractured root. B, Resorbed root. C, Incompletely formed root.

If a tooth fragments or a filling becomes detached, all loose foreign bodies must be removed from the oral cavity before any further attempt is made to extract the tooth. The problem is assessed, and if the operator feels sure that the extraction can be completed he should proceed. If he feels that it cannot be completed on this occasion he should stop, and postpone the extraction until circumstances are such that it can be completed. *If the dental pulp is exposed it must be removed* (*see* p. 69).

As each tooth is extracted it should be examined to ensure that it is complete before being placed in a receptacle. Care should be taken to see that it does not stick to the forceps and thus be conveyed back to the mouth. *Fig.* 94 and *Fig.* 54, p. 33 illustrate the difference between a fractured root and a resorbed one. The fractured surface is flat and shiny and the pulp canal is clearly visible, while the surface of a resorbed root is roughened and appears matt.

When the extractions have been completed and the sockets squeezed, all excess blood and saliva are removed from the mouth by either suction or swabbing. Administration of the anaesthetic agent is stopped and the prop removed from the mouth, but the pack is left in situ and the patient's head pulled forwards to lessen the risk of blood being inhaled. The teeth and roots are carefully examined and their number checked. When the patient has regained consciousness the pack is re-moved and he is encouraged to spit out the blood and saliva into a kidney dish. After clean folded gauze packs have been placed on the sockets, the patient is in-structed to bite upon them, and is then assisted to a recovery room in either a wheel-chair or in the manner illustrated in *Fig*. 95. With this kind of support the patient is under control, for if he either stumbles or falls he can be gently lowered to the floor without any risk of damaging himself. In the recovery room he may either sit on a chair or lie on his side upon a couch, depending upon his general condition, until he has fully recovered from the effects of the anaes-thetic. The length of the recovery period varies between individual patients and is influenced by the type and amount of anaesthetic agent employed and the dura-tion for which it was administered. The patient must have recovered completely from the effects of anaesthesia and have stopped bleeding before he is discharged.

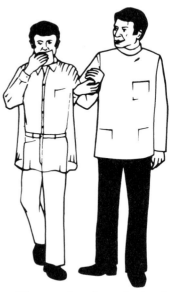

Fig. 95.—A patient who has just recovered from a general anaesthetic being assisted to a recovery room.

Special Apparatus.—Every dental surgery in which extractions are regularly performed under general anaesthesia should be equipped with an efficient suction apparatus. Many types are available (*Fig*. 96). Intelligent use of the sucker not only helps the operator, but also reduces the risk of blood being inhaled or causing laryngeal spasm. A tracheostomy set should always be kept sterile and ready for use in an emergency.

A surgical tray (*Fig*. 97) should be laid out, sterile and ready for use whenever extractions are being performed. The extraction of resistant teeth and retained roots (*see* pp. 68, 80) is facilitated if all the instruments needed are sterile and ready to hand, and vital minutes will be saved when difficulty is encountered under general anaesthesia in the dental chair.

Co-operation between the Operator and the Anaesthetist.—There is no branch of surgery calling for closer co-operation between the surgeon and the anaesthetist than the extraction of teeth under general anaesthesia in the dental chair. Each must understand precisely what is required of him and

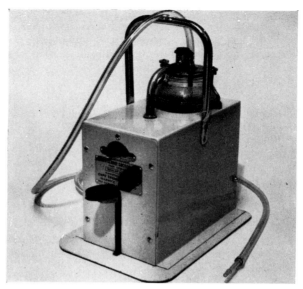

Fig. 96.—Smith Clarke foot-operated suction apparatus.

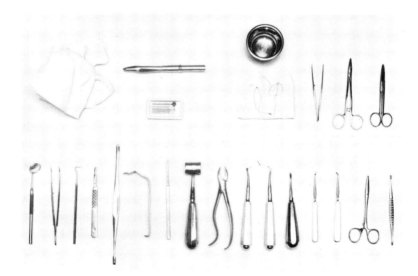

Fig. 97.—The contents of a surgical tray.

how he can best aid his colleague. The main task of the dental anaesthetist is the preservation of an unobstructed airway. He supports the mandible and listens to every breath. In addition to doing this he supports and turns the patient's head to facilitate the extraction and attempts to anticipate any assistance that the dental surgeon may require. If the operator desires co-operation of this order he must use this form of anaesthesia with discretion, tell the anaesthetist precisely what surgery is to be performed and the method he proposes to employ. The anaesthetist must also be told if a change of sides will be required and given an estimate of the duration of the operation. This estimate should allow ample time for the operation to be completed, even if it proves a little more difficult than at first anticipated.

The operator can assist the anaesthetist by supporting the mandible especially when extracting lower teeth, and ensuring that the tongue is not pushed backwards by either his left hand or the mouth pack. *If the anaesthetist asks the operator to stop operating he must do so immediately,* provided that no tooth or other foreign body is left lying free in the oral cavity. A skilled dental anaesthetist will only make such a request if it is absolutely necessary, and in such circumstances there is usually no time for either delay or debate. Sometimes the patient may vomit during either the induction or recovery stage of anaesthesia. In these circumstances the anaesthetist will hold the head forwards and the operator should suck or mop out the mouth and oropharynx.

Abscesses.—General anaesthesia in the dental chair is often used to facilitate the extraction of abscessed teeth and/or the drainage of the abscess. If the infection is in the floor of the mouth this method should not be used because of the risk of oedema of the glottis. In these circumstances the patient should be admitted to hospital if an anaesthetic is required.

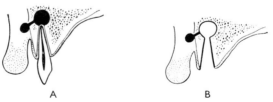

A   B

Fig. 98.—Sagittal section of an abscessed incisor. A, The pus has tracked into the labial sulcus. B, The removal of the tooth drains the intra-bony lesion, but not the pus in the soft tissues.

Removal of the tooth gives drainage to any abscess enclosed within the bone. If fluctuation, induration, or tenderness is present in the soft tissues, extraction of the tooth alone never gives sufficient drainage. The soft tissues must be incised adequately even if pus comes down the socket, for this pus will come from the intra-bony lesion only (*Fig.* 98). An incision must be made through the mucous membrane overlying the pus in the labial or buccal sulcus. The incision should be parallel to the alveolar ridge and at least 1·3 cm. (½ in.) in length. The closed blades of a pair of sinus forceps are thrust into the abscess and then opened, liberating the pus (*Fig.* 99). This method of opening an abscess ensures that no blood-vessel or nerve is damaged and is called *Hilton's method.* The postoperative use of a hot saline mouth-bath (*see* p. 39) usually ensures that the incision stays open as long as drainage is required.

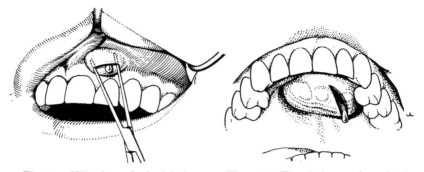

Fig. 99.—Hilton's method of drain-   Fig. 100.—The drainage of a palatal
         ing an abscess.   abscess.

When opening palatal abscesses it is necessary to make the incisions anteroposteriorly parallel to the nerves and blood-vessels in an attempt to minimize the risk of damage to these structures. In many instances it is best to remove an ellipse of tissue to ensure that the incision line is not sealed as the tongue moulds the mucoperiosteum to the palatal vault (*Fig.* 100). In this site the inflamed and thickened soft tissues often take several days to return to their normal shape and size.

Any instrument used during the extraction of an abscessed tooth or the drainage of an abscess must not be used again when working in an uninfected area of the same patient. If a virulent acute intra-oral infection is present it is best to limit the amount of surgery to that required to deal with the infection.

CHAPTER V

COMPLICATIONS OF TOOTH EXTRACTION

THE complications of tooth extraction are many and varied and some may occur even when the utmost care is exercised. Others are avoidable if a plan of campaign, designed to deal with difficulties diagnosed during a careful preoperative assessment, is implemented by an operator who adheres to sound surgical principles during the extraction.

POSSIBLE COMPLICATIONS

Failure to:—
    Secure anaesthesia
    Remove the tooth with either forceps or elevators
Fracture of:—
    Crown of tooth being extracted
    Roots of tooth being extracted
    Alveolar bone
    Maxillary tuberosity
    Adjacent or opposing tooth
    Mandible
Dislocation of:—
    Adjacent tooth
    Temporomandibular joint
Displacement of a root:—
    Into the soft tissues
    Into the maxillary antrum
    Under general anaesthesia in the dental chair
Excessive haemorrhage:—
    During tooth removal
    On completion of the extraction
    Postoperatively
Damage to:—
    Gums
    Lips
    Inferior dental nerve or its branches
    Lingual nerve
    Tongue and floor of mouth
Postoperative pain due to:—
    Damage to hard and soft tissues
    'Dry socket'
    Acute osteomyelitis of the mandible
    Traumatic arthritis of the temporomandibular joint
Postoperative swelling due to:—
    Oedema
    Haematoma formation
    Infection

Trismus
The creation of an oro-antral communication
Syncope
Respiratory arrest
Cardiac arrest
Anaesthetic emergencies

Failure to secure anaesthesia is usually due to faulty technique or insufficient dosage of the anaesthetic agent. It is impossible to extract teeth well unless both the operator and the patient have complete confidence in the anaesthesia under which the operation is performed. The employment of a skilled anaesthetist will ensure this when a general anaesthetic is administered, but when local anaesthesia is employed its efficacy should be tested before the extraction is started. After explaining to the patient that although he may feel pressure he should not feel any sensation of sharpness, a blunt probe

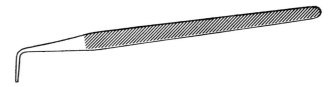

Fig. 101.—A blunt probe (Moon's pattern).

(*Fig.* 101) is pushed firmly into the gingival crevice on the buccal and lingual surfaces of the tooth to be extracted. If nothing is felt by the patient anaesthesia has been secured. If he feels pressure but not pain, analgesia has been obtained, but pain indicates that a further injection of local anaesthetic solution is required.

If a tooth *fails to yield* to the application of reasonable force applied with either *forceps* or an *elevator* the instrument should be put down and the cause of the difficulty sought (*see* p. 27). In most cases the tooth will be better removed by dissection.

Fracture of the crown of a tooth during extraction may be unavoidable if the tooth is weakened either by caries or a large restoration. However, it is often caused by the improper application of the forceps to the tooth, the blades being either applied to the crown instead of the root or root-mass, or with their long axis across that of the tooth. If the operator chooses a pair of forceps with blades which are too broad and give only 'one-point contact' (*see* p. 21) the tooth may collapse when gripped. If the forceps handles are not held firmly together the blades may slip off the root and fracture the crown of the tooth. Hurry is usually the underlying cause of all these errors of technique, which are avoidable if the operator works methodically. The exhibition of *excessive* force in an effort to overcome resistance is unwarrantable and may cause a fracture of the crown.

When coronal fracture occurs the method used to remove the retained portion of the tooth will be governed by the amount of tooth remaining and the cause of the mishap. Sometimes a further application of the forceps or elevator will deliver the tooth, and on other occasions the trans-alveolar method should be used.

When the complexity of the root-pattern of extracted teeth is considered, it is surprising, not that occasionally *roots fracture* during extraction, but that this complication does not occur more frequently. The factors causing fracture of the crown may also cause fracture of the roots and avoidance of these faults will reduce the incidence of such fracture. Although ideally all root-fragments should be removed, it is wiser to leave them in certain circumstances. *A root-apex* may be defined as a root-fragment *less than* 5 mm. *in its greatest dimension*. The removal of large amounts of bone may be necessary for the location and removal of such an apex. In healthy patients retained apices of vital teeth seldom give trouble and in most cases they should be left unless they are in such a position that they are liable to become exposed when dentures are worn or symptoms supervene. The extraction of the apical one-third of the palatal root of a maxillary molar involves the removal of a large amount of alveolar bone and may be complicated by the displacement of the fragment into the maxillary antrum or the creation of an oro-antral communication (*see* pp. 74, 81). Such fragments are better left undisturbed in the vast majority of cases. If removal is indicated it should be preceded by radiographic examination and performed by an experienced operator using the trans-alveolar method. Whenever it is decided to leave a root-fragment in situ the patient must be informed and the particulars of the retained root entered in the patient's records.

When a tooth fractures during extraction the dental surgeon should try to ascertain the reason by clinical, and in some cases radiographic, means. Examination of the portion of the tooth which has been delivered often provides a useful guide to both the size and position of the retained fragment. Then he should estimate the time and facilities required to complete the extraction. If either one or both of these requirements is not available, he should not attempt to deliver the retained portion, but should remove any exposed pulpal tissue and cover the fragments with a zinc oxide and oil of cloves dressing into which cotton-wool fibres have been incorporated. Arrangements should then be made for removal of the fragments by himself or a colleague under conditions which ensure success. After-pain is seldom a feature of such incidents if this policy is pursued and the supporting tissues have not been lacerated by hurried, clumsy, and ineffectual attempts to complete the operation.

Fracture of the alveolar bone is a common complication of tooth extraction, and examination of extracted teeth reveals alveolar fragments adhering to a number of them. This may be due to the accidental inclusion of alveolar bone within the forceps blades or to the configuration of roots, the shape of the alveolus, or to pathological changes in the bone itself. The extraction of canines is frequently complicated by fracture of the labial plate, especially if the alveolar bone has been weakened by extraction of the lateral incisor and/or the first premolar prior to the removal of the canine. If these three teeth are to be extracted at one visit, the incidence of fracture of the labial plate will be reduced if the canine is removed first.

It is advisable to remove any alveolar fragment which has lost over one-half of its periosteal attachment, by gripping it with haemostatic forceps and dissecting off the soft tissues with a periosteal elevator, a Mitchell trimmer, or a Cumine scaler.

Fracture of the maxillary tuberosity. Occasionally, during the extraction of an upper molar, the supporting bone and maxillary tuberosity are felt to move with the tooth. This accident is usually due to the invasion of the tuberosity by the antrum (*Fig.* 102), which is common when an isolated maxillary molar is present, especially if the tooth is overerupted. Pathological gemination between an erupted maxillary second molar and an unerupted maxillary third molar is a rare predisposing cause. When fracture occurs (*Fig.* 102 A, B) the forceps should be discarded and a large buccal mucoperiosteal flap raised. The fractured tuberosity and the tooth should then be freed from the palatal soft tissues by blunt dissection and lifted from the wound (*Fig.* 102 C). The soft-tissue flaps are then apposed with mattress sutures (*Fig.* 102 D) which evert the edges and are left in situ for at least 10 days. *Fig.* 102 E shows a typical end-result.

If this complication occurs in one maxilla the patient should be warned that it is liable to complicate a similar extraction performed on the other side of the mouth. Only if a preoperative radiograph reveals the possibility is it possible to reduce the risk of fracture of the tuberosity by extracting the tooth by careful dissection.

Fracture of an adjacent or opposing tooth during extraction can be avoided. Careful preoperative examination will reveal whether a tooth adjacent to that to be extracted is either carious, heavily restored, or in the line of withdrawal. If the tooth to be extracted is an abutment tooth, the bridge should be divided with a vulcarbo or diamond disk before extraction. Caries and loose or over-hanging fillings should be removed from an adjacent tooth and a temporary dressing inserted before the extraction. No force should be applied to any adjacent tooth during an extraction, and other teeth should not be used as a fulcrum for an elevator unless they are to be extracted at the same visit (*see* p. 31).

Opposing teeth may be either chipped or fractured if the tooth being extracted yields suddenly to uncontrolled force and the forceps strike them. Careful controlled extraction technique prevents this accident.

Under general anaesthesia, teeth other than the one being extracted may be damaged by the injudicious use of gags and props. The presence of heavily restored or loose teeth, crowns or bridges should be noted and brought to the attention of the anaesthetist. Such teeth should be avoided when props or gags are inserted. If possible mouth gags should not be used (*see* p. 62). Gags and props must either be placed under direct vision, or, if inserted by an anaes-thetist standing behind the patient, should be guided into place by the operator.

Fracture of the mandible may complicate tooth extraction if excessive or incorrectly applied force is used, or pathological changes have weakened the

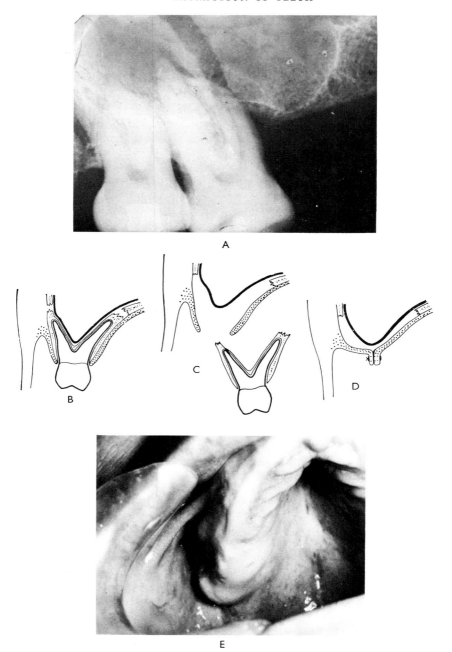

Fig. 102.—The surgical treatment of a fractured tuberosity. *See text for description.*

jaw. Excessive force should never be used to extract teeth. If a tooth does not yield to moderate pressure the reason should be sought and remedied.

The mandible may be weakened by senile osteoporosis and atrophy, osteo-myelitis, previous therapeutic irradiation, or such osteodystrophies as osteitis deformans, fibrous dysplasia, or fragilitas ossium. Unerupted teeth, cysts, hyperparathyroidism, or tumours may also predispose to fracture. In the presence of one of these conditions, extraction should be attempted only after careful clinical and radiographic assessment and the construction of splints preoperatively. The patient should be informed before operation of the possibility of mandibular fracture, and should this complication occur treatment must be instituted at once. For these reasons such cases are best dealt with in specialist oral surgery centres. If a fracture occurs in the dental surgery, extra-oral support (*see Fig.* 104) should be applied and the patient referred immediately to a hospital where facilities for treatment exist.

Dislocation of an adjacent tooth during extraction is an avoidable accident. The causes are similar to those giving rise to a fracture of an adjacent tooth and are detailed on page 70. Even during the correct use of an elevator (*see* p. 34)

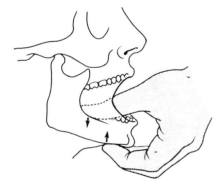

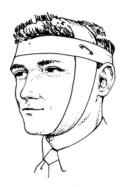

Fig. 103.—The reduction of a dislocation of the mandible. *See text for explanation.*

Fig. 104.—Extra-oral support for the mandible. The material should be of a variety which does not stretch and the vertical component must be applied as far back on the mandible as is possible.

some pressure is transmitted to the adjacent tooth through the interdental septum. For this reason an elevator should not be applied to the mesial surface of a first permanent molar, because the smaller second premolar may be dislodged from its socket. During elevation a finger should be placed upon the adjacent tooth to support it and enable any force transmitted to it to be detected.

Dislocation of the temporomandibular joint occurs readily in some patients and a history of recurrent dislocation should never be disregarded. This complication of mandibular extractions can usually be prevented if the lower jaw is supported during extraction. The support given to the jaw by the left hand of the operator should be supplemented by that given by the anaesthetist or an assistant pressing upwards with both hands beneath the angles of the mandible.

Dislocation may also be caused by the injudicious use of gags. If dislocation occurs it should be reduced immediately. The operator stands in front of the patient and places his thumbs intra-orally on the external oblique ridges lateral to any mandibular molars which are present and his fingers extra-orally under the lower border of the mandible (*Fig.* 103). Downward pressure with the thumbs and upward pressure with the fingers reduce the dislocation. If treatment is delayed muscle-spasm may make reduction impossible, except under general anaesthesia. The patient should be warned not to open his mouth too widely or to yawn for a few days postoperatively, and an extra-oral support to the joint should be applied (*Fig.* 104) and worn until tenderness in the affected joint subsides.

Displacement of a root into the soft tissues is usually the result of ineffectual attempts to grip the root when visual access is inadequate. This complication can be avoided if the operator attempts to grasp roots only under direct vision.

A root displaced into the antrum is usually that of a maxillary premolar or molar and is most often the palatal root. The presence of a large antrum is a predisposing factor, but the incidence of this complication would be greatly reduced if the following simple rules were observed:—

1. Never apply forceps to a maxillary cheek tooth or root unless sufficient of its length is exposed, both palatally and buccally, to allow the blades to be applied under direct vision.

2. Leave the apical one-third of the palatal root of a maxillary molar if it is retained during forceps extraction unless there is a positive indication for removing it.

3. Never attempt to remove a fractured maxillary root by passing instruments up the socket. If removal is indicated, raise a large mucoperiosteal flap and remove enough bone to permit an elevator to be inserted above the broken surface of the root, so that all the force applied to the root tends to move it downwards and away from the antrum.

Any previous history of antral involvement should not be disregarded, for it is probable that the patient has large maxillary sinuses. If a root is displaced into the antrum the patient must be referred to either an oral surgeon or an otorhinolaryngologist, after the freshly created oro-antral communication has been repaired and covered (*see* p. 81).

Displacement of a root into either the antrum or the soft tissues occurs more frequently under general anaesthesia in the dental chair than under local anaesthesia. If a *root is lost while teeth are being extracted under general anaesthesia*, the anaesthetic should be stopped immediately and the patient's head brought forwards. After the cough reflex has returned the mouth is examined and the pack carefully removed and inspected. If proper safeguards have been taken the root is found in the pack in most instances, but if the root cannot be located after removal of the pack, radiographs should be taken of both the socket and the chest. The latter film is taken to ensure that the root has not passed into the bronchi. Should the root be revealed lying in a bronchus, the patient must immediately be referred to a hospital where it can be removed by bronchoscopy before either a lung abscess or atelectasis supervenes. If the root is not located the patient should be given an appointment for examination in 3 days. He should be instructed to attend hospital immediately if he develops either a temperature, cough, or chest pain.

Excessive haemorrhage may complicate the extraction of teeth. Inquiries should be made to elicit any previous history of bleeding before an extraction is undertaken. If a patient states that he bleeds excessively full details should be obtained of any previous haemorrhagic episode. Particular note should be taken of the time relationship of the onset of bleeding to the extraction, the duration and amount of haemorrhage, and the measures required to combat it. A family history of bleeding is of great importance. Any patient with a history which suggests the presence of a haemorrhagic diathesis should be

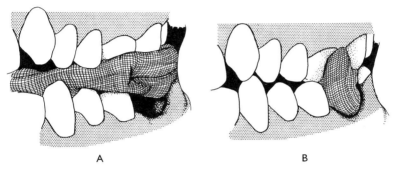

A   B

Fig. 105.—The arrest of postoperative bleeding. A, The gauze has not been placed on the socket margins and therefore it cannot aid haemostatis. B, The gauze roll is positioned correctly.

referred to a haematologist for investigation before the extractions are undertaken. If a patient has a history of previous post-extraction haemorrhage, it is wise to limit the number of teeth extracted on the first visit, to suture the soft tissues, and to observe the postoperative progress. If nothing untoward occurs the amount of surgery undertaken at succeeding visits can be increased gradually.

Sometimes constant oozing of blood *during the operation* obscures vision and makes the extraction difficult. This can be dealt with by swabbing with gauze packs or by the use of a sucker. To be of value in oral surgery the sucker should have a pressure of 0·14 kg. per sq. cm. (20 lb. per sq. in.) and should be handled by an assistant trained in its correct use. More severe bleeding can be controlled by pressure on a hot (50° C.) normal saline pack held in position for a *timed* 2 minutes. A sucker should be used to remove excess saline from the pack. Rarely, the bleeding is due to a larger vessel and in these circumstances the vessel should be picked up and clamped with a haemostat. Bleeding may be troublesome when working under general anaesthesia if oxygenation is insufficient. The vasoconstrictor present in local anaesthetic solutions usually ensures a dry operative field, and thus aids surgery.

When the *extraction is completed* the patient should be allowed to rinse the mouth with a bland mouthwash *once*. A firm gauze roll should then be placed upon the socket (*Fig.* 105) and the patient asked to bite upon it for a few minutes. If the haemorrhage is not controlled within 10 minutes, a horizontal mattress suture should be inserted into the mucoperiosteum to control the haemorrhage (*see below*).

Most patients who return complaining of *postoperative haemorrhage* are accompanied by anxious relatives or friends and it is essential to separate the patient from these well-intentioned, but unhelpful, companions. Until the patient has been taken to the dental surgery and the persons accompanying him asked to remain in the waiting room, it will be quite impossible either to reassure or treat him satisfactorily. After seating the patient comfortably in the dental chair and covering his clothes with a protective waterproof apron, the dental surgeon should examine the mouth in order to determine the site and amount of haemorrhage. Almost invariably an excess of blood-clot will be seen in the bleeding area and this should be grasped in a piece of gauze and removed. A firm gauze pack should then be placed upon the socket and the patient instructed to bite upon it. If tannic acid powder is placed upon the portion of the pack adjacent to the bleeding socket it will help to arrest the haemorrhage. In most instances it will be advisable to insert a suture into the mucoperiosteum, under local anaesthesia, to control the haemorrhage. An interrupted horizontal mattress suture is best suited to this purpose and should be inserted across the socket as soon as possible. The object of suturing is *not* to close the socket by approximating the soft tissues over it, but to tense the mucoperiosteum over the underlying bone so that it becomes ischaemic. In the vast majority of cases, the bleeding arises not in the bony socket but from the soft tissues surrounding it and is stopped by the procedure described above. The patient should be instructed to bite upon a gauze pack for 5 minutes following the insertion of a suture. Should these measures fail to control the haemorrhage, either gelatin or fibrin foam may be tucked into the socket and a composition block moulded over the area. After the block has been placed in situ (*Fig.* 106) and an extra-oral support provided, the patient should be referred to the nearest hospital for further treatment. In most cases the haemorrhage will have been arrested by simple measures and it is prudent to re-examine the patient after he has walked about before discharging him with instructions to carry out such measures as those detailed on page 39. The mouth tastes unpleasant after a dental haemorrhage, but repeated rinsing promotes bleeding and should be avoided. The oral cavity should be cleaned carefully with gauze soaked in cold water, special attention being paid to the tongue. This simple procedure adds greatly to the patient's comfort.

Damage to the gum can be avoided by careful selection of forceps and good technique. Should gum adhere to a tooth being delivered from its socket it should be carefully dissected from the tooth with either a scalpel or scissors before any further attempts to deliver the tooth are made.

The *lower lip* may be crushed between the handles of the forceps and the anterior teeth if sufficient care is not taken. The skilled use of the operator's left hand should ensure that the lip is out of harm's way. Extra care is required when maxillary teeth are being extracted under general anaesthesia. The lips may be burned if instruments are not allowed to cool before use after being sterilized.

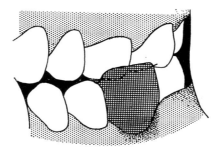

Fig. 106.—The use of a composition block for haemostasis.

If the tooth or root is in an intimate relationship with the *inferior dental nerve*, damage can be prevented or minimized only by preoperative radiographic diagnosis and careful dissection. The *mental nerve* may be damaged either during the removal of lower premolar roots or by acute inflammation in the tissues around it. If the nerve is protected by a metal retractor during operation, and bone removal is maximal mesially to a first premolar root and distally to a second premolar root, impairment of labial sensation will be avoided altogether or be minimal and transient.

The *lingual nerve* may be damaged either by a traumatic extraction of a lower molar in which the lingual soft tissues are trapped in the forceps, or by being caught up with the bur during the removal of bone. A metal retractor should be used to protect adjacent soft tissues from harm whenever a bur is in use.

The *tongue and floor of the mouth* should not be damaged during tooth extraction if care is taken during the application of forceps and the use of elevators. These mishaps occur most commonly under general anaesthesia, the soft tissues either being crushed in the forceps or between the teeth and the blades of a mouth gag. Effective use of the left hand prevents these accidents. If the operator uses an elevator without proper control he may slip and drive the instrument into either the tongue or the floor of the mouth. The tongue is very vascular and profuse bleeding may follow such an injury. This haemorrhage can be controlled by pulling the tongue forward and by the insertion of sutures. A surgical second opinion should be sought in all such cases.

The *postoperative pain* due to *traumatized hard tissues* may be from bruising of bone during instrumentation or from allowing a bur to overheat during bone removal. Avoidance of these errors of technique and attention to the smoothing of sharp bone-edges and socket toilet eliminate this cause of after-pain. *Soft tissues* may be damaged in several ways. An incision which passes through only one layer of the gingiva may lead to the mucous layer being separated from the periosteum, with the formation of a ragged flap which heals slowly. If a flap is too small, much traumatic retraction may be required to secure access, and if the soft tissues are not properly protected they may become entangled with a bur (*see* p. 44). All these errors of technique and their

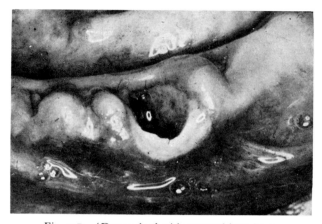

Fig. 107.—'Dry socket' with exposed bare bone.

sequelae are preventable, but unfortunately the condition known as '*dry socket*' is not. This clinical entity is a localized osteitis involving either the whole or a part of the condensed bone lining a tooth socket, the lamina dura. The condition is characterized by an acutely painful tooth socket containing bare bone and broken-down blood-clot (*Fig.* 107). The aetiology is obscure, but many predisposing causes have been noted. Infection of the socket occurring either before, during, or after the extraction may be an exciting factor, yet many abscessed and infected teeth are extracted without a 'dry socket' occurring. Although it is true that the condition may follow the use of excessive force during an extraction this is not always the case, and the complication may occur after very easy extractions. Many authorities feel that the vasoconstrictor in local anaesthetic solutions may predispose to 'dry socket' by interfering with the blood-supply of the bone, and they point out that the condition occurs more frequently under local than general anaesthesia. Nevertheless, 'dry sockets' may follow extractions performed under general anaesthesia, especially if they are clumsily performed. The incidence may be influenced by the fact that many dental surgeons perform their more difficult extractions under local anaesthesia. Vasoconstrictors are not the basic cause of the lesion, but they are a contributory factor. Mandibular extractions are complicated by the development of a 'dry socket' more frequently than maxillary extractions. The mandible has much more dense bone and is less vascular than the maxilla. Lower teeth are usually more difficult to extract than upper teeth and gravity ensures that mandibular sockets become contaminated with food debris. While it is probable that a combination of two or more of these predisposing factors makes the occurrence of a 'dry socket' more likely, it is impossible to forecast preoperatively which extractions will

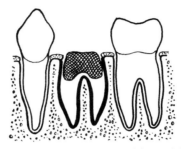

Fig. 108.—A sedative dressing tucked into a 'dry socket'.

be followed by this complication, and so the following measures aimed at prevention should be employed wherever possible. The teeth should be scaled and any gingival inflammation treated at least 1 week before the extraction of teeth. Only the minimum amount of local anaesthetic solution necessary should be administered, and the teeth should be removed as atraumatically as possible.

If a 'dry socket' occurs, the aim of treatment should be the relief of pain and the speeding of resolution. The socket should be irrigated with warm normal saline and all degenerating blood-clot removed. Sharp bony spurs should be either excised with rongeur forceps or smoothed with a wheel stone. A *loose dressing* composed of zinc oxide and oil of cloves on cotton-wool is *tucked into* the socket (*Fig.* 108). It must not be packed tightly in the socket or it may set hard and be very difficult to remove. Analgesic tablets and hot saline mouth-baths are prescribed and arrangements made to see the patient again in 3 days' time (*see* pp. 36 and 39). Most patients treated in this manner report relief of pain, but some require a further dressing or even chemical cauterization of the exposed bare painful bone to control the symptoms.

While zinc oxide and oil of cloves dressings relieve pain they undoubtedly delay healing. Though a pack composed of Whitehead's varnish (Pigmentum Iodoform Compositum B.P.C.) on either a pom-pom or ribbon gauze is not quite so effective in controlling pain, it can be left in situ for 2 or 3 weeks, and the socket will be found to be granulating when the dressing is removed.

A pom-pom (*Fig.* 109) is a piece of cotton-wool enclosed within an outer layer of gauze, the free edges of which are secured by means of a ligature of either dental floss or suture material. As it is often less painful to insert a pom-pom into a 'dry socket' than to place a ribbon-gauze pack, it is useful to have a number of sterile pom-poms of varying sizes available for immediate use.

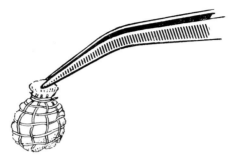

Fig. 109.—A pom-pom.

Pigmentum Iodoform Compositum B.P.C.

(Pig. Iodof. Co., Whitehead's varnish)

Benzoin, sumatra in coarse powder	44 gr. (3 g.)
Prepared storax	33 gr. (2 g.)
Balsam of Tolu	22 gr. (1·5 g.)
Iodoform	44 gr. (3 g.)
Solvent ether	to 1 fl. oz. (28·4 ml.)

1 fl. oz. (28·4 ml.) to be dispensed unless otherwise directed

Sometimes it may be difficult to differentiate between a patient afflicted with a severe 'dry socket' and one suffering from *acute osteomyelitis of the mandible*. The latter condition usually causes more general prostration and toxicity. There is marked pyrexia and pain is very severe. Often the mandible is exquisitely tender on *extra-oral* palpation, and the onset of impairment of labial sensation some hours or even days after the extraction is characteristic of acute osteomyelitis of the mandible. A patient suffering from this condition should be admitted as an emergency to a hospital where facilities for its effective treatment exist. Traumatic extraction of a lower molar under local anaesthesia in the presence of acute gingival inflammation (e.g., pericoronitis or acute ulcerative gingivitis) predisposes to acute osteomyelitis of the mandible.

Traumatic arthritis of the temporomandibular joint may complicate difficult extractions if the lower jaw is not supported. The risk of this unpleasant condition occurring can be minimized if the operator uses his left hand correctly and the anaesthetist or an assistant steadies the mandible by holding it under the angles, as described on page 25. If it is known that the patient has a history of a previous dislocation of the temporomandibular joint it is a wise precaution to get him to hold a dental prop tightly between his teeth on the contralateral side during a dental extraction.

If the soft tissues are not handled carefully during an extraction traumatic *oedema* may delay healing. The use of blunt instruments, the excessive retraction of badly designed flaps, or a bur becoming entangled in the soft tissues predispose to this condition. If sutures are tied too tightly post-operative swelling due to oedema or *haematoma* formation may cause sloughing of the soft tissues and breakdown of the suture line. Usually both conditions regress if the patient uses hot saline mouth-baths frequently for 2 or 3 days.

A more serious cause of postoperative swelling is *infection* of the wound. No effort should be spared to prevent the introduction of pathogenic micro-organisms into the wound. If the infection is mild it will often respond to the application of heat *intra-orally* by the use of frequent hot saline mouth-baths. The patient should be cautioned against applying heat extra-orally because this increases the size of the facial swelling. A hot-water bottle applied to the cheek in an effort to relieve pain is a common cause of gross swelling of the face. If fluctuation is present the pus should be evacuated before beginning antibiotic therapy (*see* p. 66). Any patient with a postoperative infection severe enough to warrant antibiotic therapy is best treated at a hospital with oral surgery facilities, especially if the swelling involves the submaxillary and sublingual tissues.

Trismus can be defined as inability to open the mouth due to muscle spasm and may complicate dental extractions. It may be caused by postoperative oedema, haematoma formation, or inflammation of the soft tissues. Patients with traumatic arthritis of the temporomandibular joints have limitation of mandibular movement. A mandibular block injection may be followed by trismus even when administered for reasons other than extraction. The treatment of trismus varies with the underlying cause. The application of intra-oral heat by means of short-wave diathermy or the use of hot saline mouth-baths gives relief in mild cases, but other patients require the administration of antibiotics or specialist treatment to relieve their symptoms.

The apices of the maxillary cheek teeth are often closely related to the antrum. Sometimes the roots are separated from the antral cavity only by the soft-tissue lining of the air sinus (*Figs.* 110 and 111 A). If this is destroyed by periapical infection or perforated during removal of a tooth or root, an *oro-antral communication* will be created (*Fig.* 111 B). If this complication is suspected the patient should be asked to grip his nose and thus occlude the nares. Then if he raises the intranasal and intra-antral pressure by attempting to blow air through his nose, in the presence of an oro-antral communication air will be heard to pass into the mouth, blood present in the socket will be seen to bubble, or a wisp of cotton-wool held over the socket will be deflected. If the test is positive or equivocal the lesion should be treated immediately. Mucoperiosteal flaps should be raised and the height of the bony socket reduced without increasing the size of the bony defect (*Fig.* 111 B). After loosely suturing the flaps across the defect with an interrupted horizontal mattress suture (*Fig.* 111 C) the repaired soft tissues and blood-clot should be supported by *covering* the area with either a quick-cure acrylic extension to an existing denture or by a base plate (*Fig.* 111 D). Alternatively, a sheet of composition impression material may be moulded to shape, cooled, trimmed, and held in place over the area, either by ligatures placed around adjacent

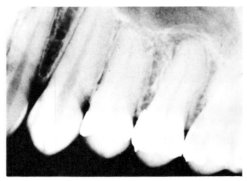

Fig. 110.—Radiograph showing a periapical area in relation to the root of a pulpless second premolar and the floor of the maxillary antrum.

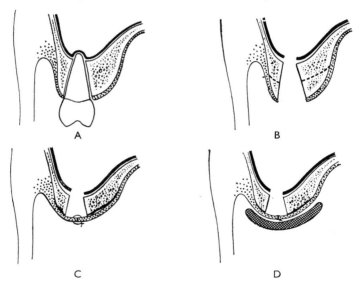

Fig. 111.—The treatment of a freshly created oro-antral communication. (*See text for explanation.*)

teeth or by sutures. The patient should then be referred for a second opinion. Under no circumstances should a patient with a suspected oro-antral communication be allowed to rinse out before the defect has been repaired, because the passage of fluid from the mouth will contaminate the air sinus with the bacterial flora of the oral cavity. The passage of instruments from the mouth into the sinus is also condemned for the same reason.

Collapse in the dental chair may occur suddenly and may or may not be accompanied by loss of consciousness. In most instances these episodes are *syncopal attacks* or 'faints' and spontaneous recovery is usual. The patient often complains of feeling dizzy, weak, and nauseated, and the skin is seen to be pale, cold, and sweating. First-aid treatment should be instituted at once and at no time should such a patient be left unattended. The head should be lowered by lowering the back of the dental chair. With some designs of chair the use of this method may entail considerable delay and in these circumstances the patient's head should be put between his knees after ensuring that his collar has been loosened. Care should be taken to *maintain the airway* and to ensure that the patient cannot fall out of the chair. *No fluids must be given by mouth until the patient is fully conscious.*

When consciousness returns a glucose drink may be given if the patient has missed a meal and is being treated under local anaesthesia. Alternatively, Spr. Ammon. Aromat. B.P.C. (Sal volatile) 3·6 ml. (1 drachm) in at least one-third of a tumblerful of water may be administered. Spontaneous recovery is usual and it is often possible to complete the extraction at the same visit.

If recovery does not occur within a few minutes of first-aid measures being instituted, the collapse is probably not of syncopal origin and oxygen should be administered and medical aid summoned. Careful note should be taken of both the type and rate of respirations, and the rate, volume, and character of the pulse. If circumstances permit, the blood-pressure should be recorded at intervals and an intravenous injection of 250 mg. of aminophylline injection B.P. may be given slowly.

If respiratory arrest occurs the skeletal muscles become flaccid and the pupils are widely dilated. The patient should be laid flat on the floor and his airway should be cleared by the removal of any appliances or foreign bodies and by pulling the mandible upwards and forwards to extend the head fully (*Fig.* 112 A). The patient's nostrils should be compressed between the operator's finger and thumb, and mouth-to-mouth resuscitation should be performed so that the chest is seen to rise every 3 or 4 seconds (*Fig.* 112 B). The efficiency of this form of resuscitation is greatly enhanced if a Brook airway (*Fig.* 113) is available and can be inserted over the tongue. Whilst he is attempting to remedy respiratory arrest the dental surgeon must check the carotid pulse and apex beat at regular intervals, for cessation of breathing may be quickly followed by cardiac arrest, which is a more sinister emergency.

Unless the circulation can be restored and maintained within 3 minutes of *cardiac arrest* occurring, irreversible brain damage may occur due to cerebral anoxia. The patient exhibits a deathly pallor and greyness, and his skin is covered with a cold sweat. The pulse and apex beat cannot be felt and the heart-sounds cannot be heard. If the patient is a child, the heart will often start beating again if the sternum is tapped sharply. When an adult is being treated the patient should be laid flat on his back on the floor. The dental

surgeon kneels at one side of his trunk and places the heel of his left hand on
the lower third of the patient's sternum. The operator then places his right
hand on the back of the heel of his left hand and presses downwards rhyth-
mically at 1-second intervals, with sufficient force to compress the heart

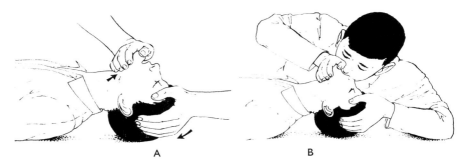

A   B

Fig. 112.—Mouth-to-mouth resuscitation. A, Extending the head to clear the
airway. B, Technique of artificial respiration. If the external nares cannot be
covered by the operator's mouth they must be compressed between his finger and
thumb.

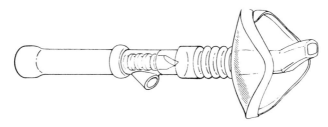

Fig. 113.—The Brook airway.

between the sternum and the vertebral column (*Fig.* 114). If an assistant is
present she should simultaneously treat the respiratory arrest in the manner
described above. When no assistance is available the dental surgeon should
perform respiratory and cardiac resuscitation alternately for periods of
20 seconds.

Prolonged resuscitation is an exhausting business and although theoretically
it should be continued until the patient's colour improves, his pupils contract,
and respiration and heart-beats are restored, an unassisted operator can only
maintain resuscitation for a limited period. This period can be greatly
prolonged if assistance is available and the individuals participating in the
resuscitation of the patient take turns at cardiac massage and mouth-to-mouth
respiration alternately.

Anaesthetic emergencies may occur despite every care being exercised.
Syncope, respiratory obstruction and arrest, and cardiac arrest may complicate

general anaesthesia, and both the anaesthetist and the operator must always be on the alert for warning signs. If collapse occurs the anaesthetic must be stopped immediately and the airway should be cleared, all packs, apparatus, and debris being removed from the mouth. The mandible and tongue should be pulled forwards, the neck extended, and the head either held downwards and forwards if the patient cannot be lifted from the chair, or upwards if he can

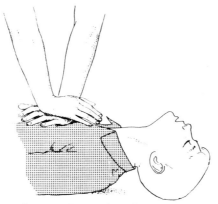

Fig. 114.—External cardiac massage.

be laid on the floor. Oxygen should be given if there is excessive contraction of the accessory muscles of respiration. If the obstruction to respiration is not relieved, either laryngotomy or tracheostomy must be performed. Should either respiratory or cardiac arrest occur it should be treated in the manner outlined above.

It is the duty of the dental surgeon to make every endeavour to avoid complications and to prevent emergencies arising. Although it is not possible to prevent them occurring completely, both their incidence and their effects can be reduced by the exercise of care and skill. Complications can only be diagnosed as soon as they occur and dealt with promptly and effectively if the possibility of their occurring has been anticipated. All too often practitioners only start thinking about emergencies and planning how to cope with them after one has arisen and exposed their inadequacies.

The dental surgeon should use a dental chair the design of which permits the patient to be quickly placed upon his back in an emergency. Otherwise an unconscious patient will have to be lifted out of the chair and on to the floor. Little purpose will be served by this exhausting manœuvre if there is insufficient free space available for the patient to be laid down and resuscitated. It is as useless to have oxygen available for use when the tubing is too short to allow the mask to be applied to the face of a supine patient, as to know which drug should be given if it and the apparatus and expertise required to administer it are not readily available.

Times of stress and crisis are ill-suited for either the acquisition of new clinical skills or the institution of a search in the telephone directory for the numbers of doctors or hospitals. For these reasons every dental surgeon should try to foresee possible emergencies and prepare for them. He should instruct each member of his staff in the role that he or she will play when a crisis occurs and should hold regular practices and checks on his emergency equipment and arrangements.

APPENDIX

EVERY dental surgeon has his favourite instruments and this results in a bewildering array of patterns being available for use. The student learning to remove teeth should endeavour to acquire proficiency in the use of a limited number of instruments in the first stages. This objective is best achieved by utilizing a basic kit of instruments and, whilst different teachers would probably have differing views on the composition of such a kit, most of them would agree that stainless-steel instruments should be used as far as is practicable.

The standard kit employed by the author for this purpose can conveniently be divided into two parts. The forceps, elevators, gags, and props are used initially and only when the technique of intra-alveolar extraction has been mastered is the student introduced to the techniques and instruments employed in trans-alveolar extraction.

The kit comprises:—

DENTAL EXTRACTION FORCEPS

For Permanent Teeth	Pattern Number
Lower root (fine)	74N
Lower root (heavy)	137
Lower full molar	73
Upper straight (fine)	29
Upper straight (heavy)	2
Upper premolar (Read)	76S
Upper premolar (fine)	147
Upper full molar (right and left)	94 and 95
Upper bayonet	101

For Deciduous Teeth	
Upper straight	163
Upper root	159
Upper full molar	157
Lower root	162
Lower full molar	160

ELEVATORS

Warwick James' pattern (right and left)
Cryer's pattern 30/31 (right and left)
Lindo Levien's pattern (large, medium, and small)

Mouth gag with Ferguson ratchet
McKesson mouth props (set of three)

OTHER SURGICAL INSTRUMENTS

Cheek retractor (Kilner's pattern)
Flap retractor (Austin's pattern)
Flap retractor (Bowdler Henry's pattern)
Scalpel handle No. 3
Scalpel blades No. 15
Mitchell's trimmer or Cumine's scaler
Waugh's mouse-toothed forceps
Periosteal elevator (Howarth's pattern)
Ash surgical burs (Toller's pattern)
Chisels (French's pattern), 5 mm., 7 mm., 9 mm., 11 mm. in width
Mallet (Weiss pattern) B 179 7½ in.
Curved artery forceps (Mosquito pattern)
Syringe (for irrigation)
Needle-holders (Kilner's pattern)
Suture needles (Lane's No. 22 half-circle cutting)
Mersilk, No. 000
Ash's No. 5S alveolotomy shears
Rongeur forceps (Ash's No. 3)
Ash's 'acrylic tools' (Nos. 6, 8, 20R)
Dental mirror, straight probe, and College tweezers
Straight dental handpiece, Kavo

It is also wise to keep certain other equipment and materials available such as:—

a. For Treatment Purposes

Whitehead's varnish
Thrombin
Gelfoam
Prilocaine 3 per cent with felypressin
Neb. Ephedrine 1 per cent in normal saline
Tinct. Benzoin. Co. inhalations
Carbolized resin
Pom-poms
Tannic acid powder
Material for chin supports

b. For Use in Emergencies

Most of the emergencies which are likely to occur in the dental surgery can be dealt with effectively by the prompt application of the basic methods of resuscitation without recourse to drug therapy. Carefully planned arrangements and well designed equipment can facilitate resuscitation in the following ways:—

Requirement	Achieved by
1. Patient in supine position	Use of dental chair designed to effect this quickly, and/or surgery design permitting the patient to be laid on floor with ease
2. A patent airway	Efficient suction apparatus (0·14 kg. per sq. cm., 20 lb./sq. in.) · Guedel's airways · Oxygen — Readily available
3. Artificial respiration	Brook airway · Inflating bellows (Ambu, Porten) · Training all of members of staff
4. External cardiac massage	Training of all members of staff

On occasions the use of the following drugs may prove to be life saving:

1. *When given intravenously:*
   50 per cent dextrose solution 20–100 ml. ampoules.
   Hydrocortisone hemisuccinate 100 mg. in 2 ml.
   Phentolamine methane sulphonate (Rogitine) 5 mg.

2. *When injected directly into the heart:*
   10 per cent calcium chloride solution 5 ml.

3. *When given intramuscularly;*
   0·1 per cent (1 : 1000) adrenaline solution 1 ml.

and so—

Sterile disposable syringes (2·5 ml. and 10 ml. side-nozzle)
Sterile No. 1 needles—

should be kept in a handy place.

INDEX